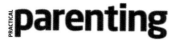

PRACTICAL **parenting**

labour & birth

all your questions answered

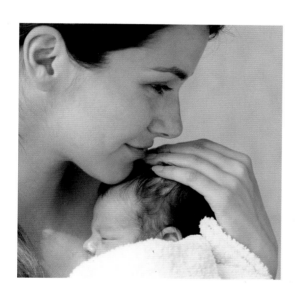

Labour & Birth has been produced in association with Practical Parenting (an IPC Media Limited publication)

Practical Parenting ® is a registered trademark of IPC Media

First published in Great Britain in 2006 by Hamlyn, a division of Octopus Publishing Group Ltd 2–4 Heron Quays, London E14 4JP

ISBN-13: 978-0-600-61481-4
ISBN-10: 0-600-61481-6

A CIP catalogue record for this book is available from the British Library

Printed and bound in China

10 9 8 7 6 5 4 3 2 1

Notes

This book is not intended as a substitute for personal medical advice. The reader should consult a physician in all matters relating to health and particularly in respect of any symptoms which may require diagnosis or medical attention. While the advice and information are believed to be accurate and true at the time of going to press, neither the author nor the publisher can accept any legal responsibility or liability for errors or omissions that may be made.

Some of the material in this book has appeared in *Practical Parenting Your Pregnancy Week by Week* (2006) and *Practical Parenting Pregnancy & Birth* (Gill Thorn, 1995), also published by Hamlyn.

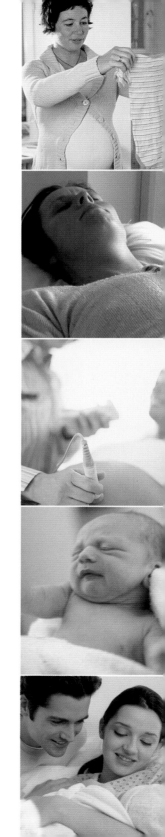

contents

introduction

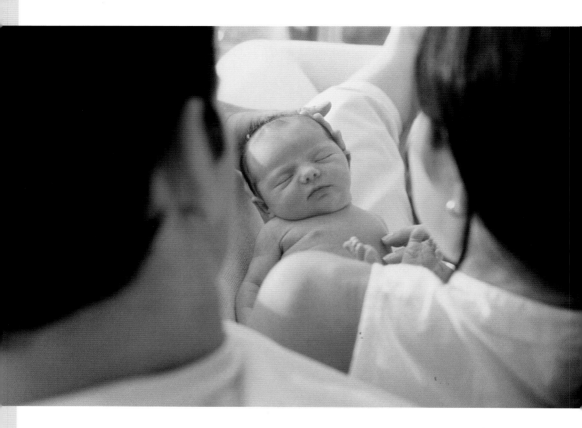

The birth of your baby may be the culmination of not only nine months of pregnancy, but of months or years of planning and dreaming. When you first found out you were pregnant it may have seemed very unreal, too huge a concept to take on board, but it is surprising how quickly the months can pass. Before the big day, it is best to gather as much information as possible, so you can make your own decisions about your care. One thing is certain: put a group of mothers together and they'll all have had very different experiences of labour and birth.

Taking control

As you approach your last month of pregnancy, you will doubtless have many questions to ask. What if my baby is early or late? Will I cope with the pain? Can I have a home birth? In my role as a midwife I am often asked about these and many other aspects of labour and birth. Remember that your midwife is there to care for you and your baby, to share information and reassure you and, importantly, to be your advocate, helping you to achieve the birth experience that you would like.

If you are well informed and can make your own decisions, your experience of labour and birth should be positive. The key to it all is relaxation and taking control, and that is the message of this book. Produced in association with *Practical Parenting* magazine, this book is a comprehensive guide to labour and birth, in an accessible question-and-answer format. Reading and learning about what might happen will give you the confidence to deal with any situation that might arise. It is important to take ownership of your pregnancy and birth – nobody will 'deliver' your baby, like a parcel; you will 'give birth', so believe in yourself and your body's ability to do so.

From packing your hospital bag to changing the first nappy, this book includes detailed advice from a team of midwives and other experts. The advice covers all aspects of labour and birth, including hospital and home births, options for medical and natural pain relief, best labour positions and looking after a baby during the first few days after the birth.

Not all births are straightforward, so you will find that this book also answers questions about assisted birth and caesarean sections, premature or overdue babies, multiple births and special-care babies. There are several

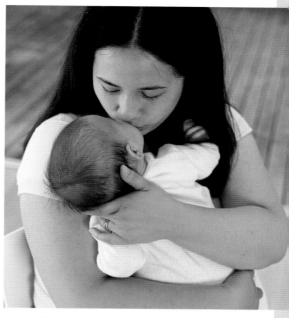

Above: A positive birth experience, in which the mother feels in control, can help the bonding process.

special features – on water birth, for example, or monitoring the baby – as well as a number of 'real-life' accounts of labour and birth, which demonstrate how varied the experiences of different mothers can be.

As a midwife, being part of a woman's experience of pregnancy and birth has been an amazing privilege. While all births are different, I have found that a woman who has the right support and information, and who is relaxed and in control, should have a positive experience of labour and birth.

Anne Richley

Anne Richley is a community midwife and the mother of two children. She regularly provides expert advice in *Practical Parenting* magazine.

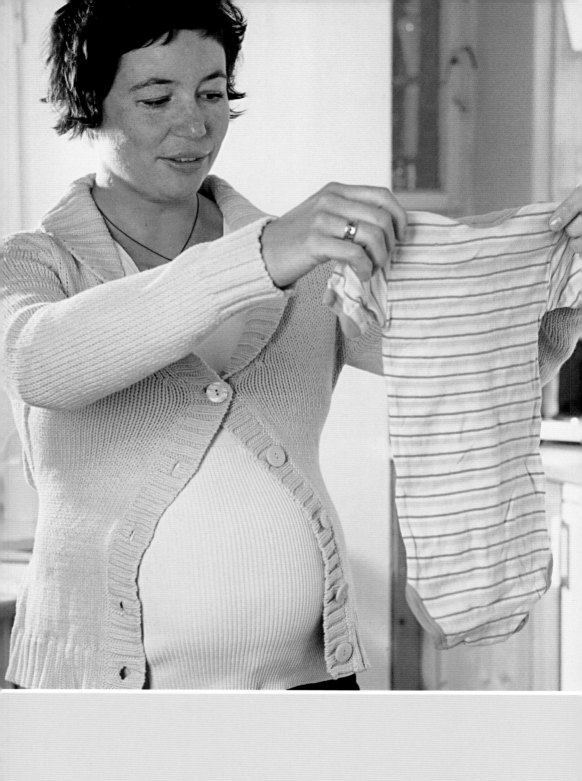

1

getting ready

Late pregnancy
You and your baby

Normal gestation is anything between 37 and 42 weeks, and you will not necessarily have the 'textbook' 40-weeks pregnancy. As you approach full term, the top of your uterus will be as high as it gets – resting just under your breastbone. When your baby's head engages you may notice that your bump drops slightly.

Your antenatal checks will be more regular now and, if you have been seeing the same staff each time, you will have built up a good relationship with the midwife and her team, so that you feel able to ask questions, seek advice or discuss any worries. In addition to the familiar procedures – checking blood pressure and testing urine – the midwife will now also assess your baby's position (see page 56).

Women often find that their 'nesting instinct' kicks in around now, and they start to prepare for the baby's birth. You may get a final burst of energy and find yourself cleaning out cupboards, washing baby clothes or wanting to decorate the baby's room. Relax once in a while for a full five minutes: sit comfortably, with your shoulders down and hands palm uppermost in your lap. Concentrate on your outward breaths because it is difficult to be tense when you are breathing out. Feel your body relaxing, like you do when you sit in a chair and sigh at the end of a busy day.

How are you sleeping?

You will probably be getting up at night, possibly several times, to empty your bladder, or you may be lying in bed awake, desperately tired with an active baby inside your uterus. There is nothing worse than lying awake in bed, thinking that you should be sleeping. If you cannot sleep, read a book or a magazine – you will feel sleepy again soon enough. On the positive side, at least insomnia prepares your body for night feeds after your baby arrives. When you are really exhausted you will sleep soundly in any position, and it pays to take a nap during the day in these last few weeks.

Five steps to getting a **good night's sleep**

There are a number of things you can do to help yourself sleep:
1 Exercise by going out for a walk for about 20 minutes each day.
2 Make sure your bedroom is neither too hot nor too cold.
3 If you sleep on your side, wedge a pillow under your bump for support.
4 Have a light snack an hour before bedtime to keep up your blood sugar levels.
5 Do not get overtired during the day – try to take a nap at some time.

Your baby's development

If this is your first baby, and he is lying in a head-down position, the head will start to descend into your pelvis at around 37 weeks. Subsequent babies often do not engage until the onset of labour, so don't worry if you are having a second baby and you don't notice your abdomen changing shape (an indication that the baby's head is engaging).

After the head has engaged, the baby's movements will be less vigorous, but he should still be active and you should still be feeling at least ten movements a day. As space becomes increasingly restricted in your uterus, your baby will be tightly curled up, with his chin tucked onto his chest and his knees drawn up to his abdomen (it is not surprising that newborn babies like to be held close and made to feel secure).

By now, all major development of your baby is complete. However, he will continue to grow in size and strength, and to lay down fat – up to 28 g (1 oz) a day. The cells in his brain will continue to multiply and develop for the first few months after birth. Your baby's appearance will not change significantly now. He is a slightly smaller version of what he will look like when he is born.

At 40 weeks your baby is fully developed. Even inside you, he is practising turning his head to one side to look for milk and sucking. At birth, major changes will take place in your baby's heart and lungs. Up until birth, the exchange of oxygen and carbon dioxide has been through the placenta. As soon as he is born and takes his first breath, the blood in his lungs will be oxygenated and he will begin to breathe normally. His rate of respiration will be about 50 breaths per minute, although it is often irregular for the first few days.

The fontanelle

The bones of your baby's skull remain soft so that they can ride over each other and mould to the shape of the birth canal. As a result, his head may be slightly pointed when he is born, and he may have some swelling either side of the head. This is only temporary. However, there will be a soft spot on the top of his head, called the fontanelle, for about 18 months, until the bones fuse together.

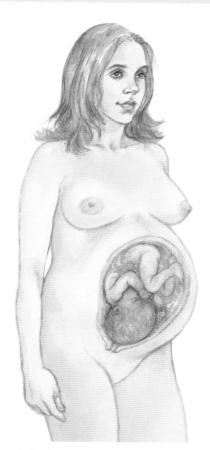

Above: At 37–40 weeks most babies are head down and ready for the birth.

Late pregnancy
How are you feeling?

Physically you may feel fit and ready for the events to come, but are you prepared mentally? There will be days when you feel excited and impatient to meet your baby and others when you are panic-stricken by the thought of labour or the responsibility of being a mother.

If this is your first baby, you may have specific concerns, such as tearing and opening your bowels during the birth, as well as less well-formulated worries. You know that it is going to

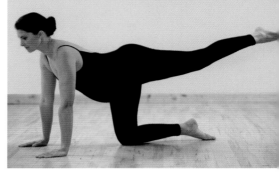

Above: Gentle exercises will help prepare your body and mind for the physical challenge to come.

hurt, but no one can tell you how much. You have no idea whether you are going to need an induction, pain relief or an assisted birth. There are so many possible scenarios that you may find it difficult to focus on them. Do not be tempted to ignore information. The more you know, the better you will feel as the big day approaches. You will be less anxious and more in control of events as they unfold.

Five steps to **taking control**

A positive state of mind is essential. No one can guarantee the perfect natural birth, but your experience will be more positive if you make the effort to prepare yourself mentally.

1 Be informed Read as much as you can about all aspects of labour and birth so that you are able to make choices and take part in the decision-making.

2 Push for the birth you want Being unhappy or uncomfortable about where and how you are expecting to go through labour and birth can have a negative influence on your experience (see Your birth plan, page 22).

3 Think positive Prepare yourself emotionally for labour and the birth. Tell yourself that you can do it and believe in your body's ability to give birth.

4 Focus on the baby Remember what it is all about – seeing your baby for the first time should be a focus for you.

5 Train your mind Practise meditation and visualization – both encourage a deep state of relaxation, which can make labour easier.

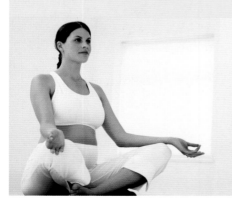

Left: Techniques of meditation and visualization can help you relax before and during labour.

Late pregnancy **Common questions**

Q Can I continue to exercise during late pregnancy?

A Exercising and staying fit should be a priority throughout your pregnancy. This will improve your circulation, help you sleep better, increase the oxygen flow to your baby, and boost your strength, stamina and suppleness. If you are not used to exercise, try something gentle, such as swimming, yoga or walking.

Q When is the best time to stop work?

A Choosing the right time to give up work is a common problem, particularly if you intend to return to work and have a limited amount of maternity leave. Many women try to make the most of their maternity leave by working as far into the pregnancy as possible. However, it can be very difficult being at home with a baby only a week or two after giving up work. Bear in mind that it is important to have some time to mentally prepare for your baby's arrival.

Q My hands and ankles have become increasingly swollen over the last few weeks. Should I be worried about this?

A Women often get a generalized swelling that includes their hands and feet and, less commonly, their face and abdomen (more common if your blood pressure is rising). This is caused by fluid retention, an increase in blood volume and a sluggish circulation, and it occurs in up to 80 per cent of pregnant women because the overall amount of fluid in the body increases during pregnancy. However, it is very important to get any

sudden change checked out by a midwife, as it could be a sign of pre-eclampsia. This complication affects one in ten pregnancies overall and one in 50 severely. It can be life-threatening to both the mother and baby if allowed to develop and progress undetected.

Q I am kept awake at night by a tingling sensation in my fingers. What is causing it?

A What you describe is carpal tunnel syndrome (CTS), which women can develop in the middle and latter part of pregnancy because of the increase in fluid. The fluid puts pressure on the median nerve in the wrist and on the carpal tunnel through which the nerve runs. The nerve becomes swollen, leading to pins and needles in the fingers and up the arm. Symptoms tend to be worse at night after the build-up of fluid during the day. Try resting your hands on your pillow when you sleep. Gentle exercise helps disperse the fluid – try circling your wrists and putting your hands in cold water. The condition usually clears up within a few weeks of the birth.

Q Should I be eating any specific foods?

A You should eat a healthy, well-balanced diet, but there is no need to 'eat for two'. It is a good idea to eat plenty of iron-rich foods, such as lean meat, leafy greens and wholegrain bread, to stock up your iron reserves. Even if you are not anaemic, you will inevitably lose a certain amount of blood during the birth. Dried fruits, such as raisins and apricots, contain iron in an easily digestible form.

Early babies

About 85 per cent of babies are born within two weeks either side of their due date. When this date is calculated from the first day of your last period, some 10 per cent (mostly first babies) are two weeks overdue. When it is estimated by ultrasound scan, only about 2 per cent of babies arrive two weeks late. If you think of 42 weeks as your due date, you will become less frustrated towards the end of your pregnancy.

'I never dreamt that our baby would be born early. We had nothing prepared but the only thing that mattered was that she was all right. The members of staff on the special-care baby unit were amazing. We will never be able to thank them enough for the care that they gave Millie, and I will never forget the day we were able to bring her home.'

Julie, mother of Millie

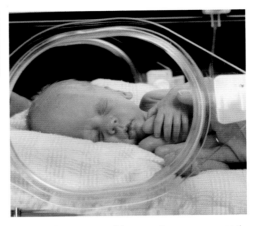

Above: Wherever possible, parents are encouraged to make physical contact with a premature baby.

Premature babies

All babies born before 37 weeks of pregnancy are deemed pre-term or premature, although a baby born at 24 weeks is obviously going to need a lot more help than one born at 36 weeks because she will still be very immature at that age.

Premature babies are more prone to infection and, unfortunately, being premature is the single biggest cause of death in babies. Although the survival rate of premature babies has increased over the last few years – and many premature babies soon catch up with their full-term peers – the number of babies born prematurely has not reduced significantly. Also there is an increased risk of disability among premature babies, particularly those born extremely early.

Coping with a premature baby

When you are not practically or emotionally prepared, the early arrival of your baby can be quite overwhelming. You may find that her condition varies from day to day, depending on how early she was born, and that there may be

Early babies **Common questions**

Q What should I do if I happen to go into labour early?

A If you notice signs of labour starting and it is three weeks or more before your due date, contact the labour ward straight away. Many babies come early without problems, but some will need specialist help. If you have several weeks to go, the hospital may try to delay your labour with drugs in order to give your baby more time to mature. Take your notes with you whenever you stay away from home and contact the nearest hospital if labour does start.

Q Why do premature babies need to be put on a mechanical ventilator?

A Many premature babies need help with their breathing because it is not until the final weeks of pregnancy that their lungs are fully mature. A mechanical ventilator may be used to push air in and out of your baby's lungs until she is able to do so herself.

Q My sister's premature baby spent his first three days in an incubator. Why was this treatment necessary?

A Small babies do not have much fat laid down and can lose heat very easily. If they get cold, they will not feed and their blood sugar level will fall. Many premature babies are therefore cared for in an incubator, where they can be kept warm.

Q Is it possible to breastfeed an early baby?

A Very small babies are unable to suck on the breast at first, but this does not mean you should abandon all hope of breastfeeding, as it has huge benefits for your baby. You can express milk, and this can be given to your baby through a tube. This also ensures that you will have a good supply of milk when your baby does get bigger and stronger, when she can then be put to the breast.

times when it is a matter of two steps forward and one step back.

You will have a vital role to play, especially if your baby is on the special-care baby unit, where she is likely to be in an incubator. This is a plastic cot with a lid and a thermostat to control the temperature. There is a port-hole through which you can touch and stroke your baby.

It is important to establish physical contact whenever possible. You should be encouraged to help with feeding and washing your baby and changing her nappy (see also Special-care babies, page 108).

Five risk factors for a **premature birth**

It is difficult to identify which women are most at risk, but certain factors are known to increase the chances of having a premature baby. These include:

1 Smoking
2 Use of recreational drugs
3 Very high caffeine intake
4 Previous premature birth
5 Previous cervical surgery

OVERDUE BABIES

Getting labour started

It can be depressing to see your due date come and go with no sign of labour, and this can seem like the longest part of pregnancy.

Although the majority of babies arrive after the due date – mostly within 14 days – waiting for the first sign of labour can feel like a very long drawn-out affair. Instead of letting yourself feel impatient and frustrated, try to focus on the last few days before your baby's arrival as a special time for you and your partner.

Nobody can say exactly when a labour is supposed to start because a 'normal' gestation is between 37 and 42 weeks. However, women are usually offered an induced labour 7–14 days after their due date. If you do not want to be induced, talk to your obstetrician or midwife. He or she should offer to monitor your baby's heartbeat at least twice a week with an electronic monitor, and to measure the fluid around your baby with ultrasound. You will also be advised to monitor your baby's movements.

Being induced

At 10–12 days overdue, your doctor will probably advise an induction (see page 72). This is because after a certain period the placenta – the source of your baby's nutrition – may stop working efficiently, and your baby may not be getting enough nourishment.

Your midwife can carry out an internal 'stretch and sweep' examination, in which she sweeps her finger around the membranes (the bag of waters around your baby). If that does not bring on labour, you will probably be asked to go into hospital for a prostaglandin pessary, which 'ripens' the cervix, so that it is soft enough to open up and make your uterus contract. Eventually, the midwife should be able to break your waters. This is no more uncomfortable than an internal examination.

If that does not start your contractions, you may be put on a drip of Syntocinon (a synthetic form of oxytoxin, a hormone that makes the uterus contract). In some cases, induction does not work and the baby is delivered by caesarean section (see page 96).

'Every day that I went past my due date felt like an extra week. The trouble was that I had not bothered arranging to do anything or go anywhere as I assumed that I would have had the baby by then. Those eight days seemed like the longest of my life!'
Betty, mother of Charlotte

Seven ways to **get labour started**

If you are past your due date there are things you can try to get labour going. If your cervix is already 'ripe', then self-help methods can help to spur things along. However, none of these methods will trigger labour unless your baby is ready to be born.

Nipple stimulation	• Use a shower attachment or breast pump to stimulate your nipples. This may encourage your body to release the hormone oxytocin, which makes your uterus contract and sets off labour. You would probably need to do this for about an hour, several times a day.
Sex	• This allows the semen to bathe the cervix, which can help to soften it and encourage labour to start. Semen is a natural source of the hormone prostaglandin, which is used in hospitals to induce labour.
Masturbation	• If neither you nor your partner feel like sex, which is not uncommon towards the end of pregnancy, masturbation can help labour. When aroused, your body releases the hormone oxytocin, which can make your uterus contract, leading to labour.
Herbal remedies	• An infusion of raspberry leaf (also available in capsule form) is reported to help ripen the cervix. Herbal remedies like these can be quite powerful, so do not drink them before 35 weeks of pregnancy in order to avoid the risk of going into labour prematurely.
Reflexology	• There is a pressure point on the foot that can stimulate contractions of the uterus, but you should consult a qualified reflexologist about this.
Walking	• Taking a long walk may encourage your baby to move in the right direction and also puts pressure on the cervix, which is good for starting labour.
Spicy foods	• If you normally eat spicy foods, they will probably have no effect, but the idea is to eat something that will loosen your bowels, which can irritate the uterus and kick-start labour. A huge bowl of fresh fruit may have the same effect!

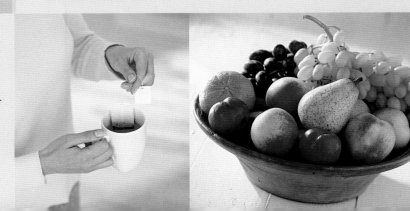

Right: An infusion of raspberry leaf may ripen the cervix and get labour started.

Far right: The bowel-loosening effect of fresh fruit can also encourage the onset of labour.

Antenatal care
What are my options?

Depending on the kind of care you want during your pregnancy and where you want to give birth (see pages 20 and 22), there are various antenatal care schemes available. Getting as much information as you can about each will help you to choose the one that is right for you.

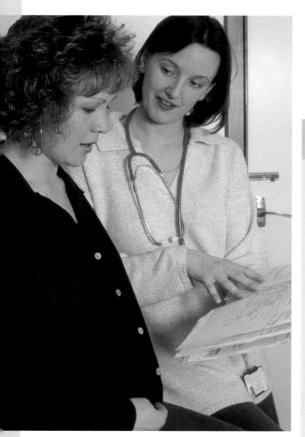

Above: Talk through the different options before deciding on your source of antenatal care.

Midwife-led care

Where care is midwife led, it is the midwives who provide all your antenatal care and, as long as your pregnancy continues to be straightforward, a midwife will also provide your labour and post-natal care. How this care is provided depends on what is available in the area where you live. Your community midwife can provide your antenatal checks, either in a clinic or in your home. You may see various midwives who are part of a team, or you may have one named midwife throughout your pregnancy. There may be a domino scheme, where your midwife accompanies you to hospital when you are in labour and discharges you some time after the birth.

Student midwives

Student midwives always work under the close supervision of a qualified member of staff, and your permission will be asked if a student wishes to be present during the birth. If it concerns you, let the midwife know or make it part of your birth plan (see page 22).

Women often imagine that there will be a crowd of students gathered in the delivery room, but this is no longer the case. At most you can expect a student midwife or student nurse who can offer additional support.

By staying with you during labour, a student midwife offers continuity of care, and this has shown to have a positive effect on a woman's ability to cope.

True story

Private antenatal care

'My first two children were born in state hospitals, but I saw a different midwife on every antenatal visit and had not met the one who delivered my children.

'I paid for a private birth with Hamish. I saw the same two midwives throughout my pregnancy, and they were with me when I gave birth, in water, after a very short labour. After the birth they cared for me for 28 days. Now I am pregnant again, I've booked a home birth with an independent midwife. It is costing a reasonable amount of money but I see it as a priority because I get antenatal appointments in my own home and my midwife treats me as an individual. Should I need to transfer to a hospital, she will come with me, and she has a contract with the hospital so she can care for me there.'

Victoria, mother of Joshua, Kitty and Hamish

Shared care

This is where antenatal care is shared between the midwife and the consultant obstetrician at the hospital or maternity unit. Shared care is usually recommended if your pregnancy falls into a 'higher risk' category – for example, if you have a complicated obstetric or medical history, are pregnant with twins or have diabetes. Your midwife will explain why this recommendation is being made but, ultimately, it is your choice.

Private care

There are some women who choose to employ an independent midwife to provide all their care. They like to be guaranteed of having the same midwife providing continuity of care throughout their pregnancy, during the birth and also post-natally. Statistically, independent midwives attend a high proportion of home births. You could also pay to see an obstetrician privately for your antenatal care, or choose to give birth in a private maternity unit.

There are several other options for private care. Some women choose to employ a post-natal maternity nurse. She will help you to establish breastfeeding, as well as answer any concerns that you might have and generally assist in building your confidence with your newborn. It is also possible to hire a night nanny to care for your baby overnight. This includes feeding your baby so that you can get some sleep, or at least a good rest. A third option is to employ a doula (see page 39), who will offer support before and during labour, as well as after the birth.

Birth choices

You have a choice when it comes to where to have your baby. The options include not only home and hospital, but also which hospital. There may be several hospitals in your area, and a range of different types of care – from birthing centres to consultant-led units – may be available.

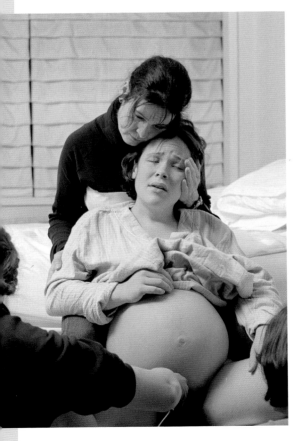

Home birth

Some women would prefer to give birth at home, where they feel comfortable and with their family close at hand, rather than in the unfamiliar, more clinical surroundings of a hospital. If your pregnancy is uncomplicated then, statistically, it is not safer to give birth in hospital (see also page 30).

Hospital (consultant unit)

These units have obstetricians on their staff, as well as all the facilities to deal with any complication during the birth. If your labour is straightforward, you will have a midwife caring for you in labour and during the birth. However, if there are any problems, an obstetrician will be available to carry out an instrumental delivery (forceps or ventouse, see page 90) or a caesarean section (see page 96).

You will also have the option of a full range of pain relief, including an epidural, which is administered by an anaesthetist (see page 50).

Midwife unit

This is usually a much smaller, often stand-alone, unit, or birthing centre, where midwives and health-care assistants provide the care. Women are encouraged to have an active birth, and a birthing pool is usually available. This type of unit is more suitable for women with uncomplicated pregnancies who do not anticipate any complications in labour.

Left: If you choose to birth at home, your midwife will provide you with one-to-one support.

Birth choices **Common questions**

Q Do I still need to visit my doctor if I am having midwife-led care?
A Whether or not you see a doctor is your choice. Most women do not need to see anyone other than their midwife.

Q What are the advantages of having my baby at home?
A If you give birth at home, you are likely to need less pain relief and will experience less intervention. You are also more likely to know the midwife who looks after you and to feel more in control throughout the birth.

Q What happens if I opt for a home birth in early pregnancy but later change my mind?
A Whatever you decide, circumstances may change during your pregnancy and influence your decision. There is no contract to sign and no one will chastise you for changing your mind.

Q Can I have a water birth?
A Water births are becoming more popular. Birthing pools offer gentle pain relief, as well as a soothing or private space in which to labour and deliver your baby. They are becoming more common in hospitals now, but policies vary on who can use them (see Water birth, page 34). Remember that, even though you may have planned a water birth, the pool may be in use when you go into labour. You should also bear in mind that you can hire your own birthing pool, either to use at home or to take to the hospital with you.

Q Do all hospitals follow the same procedure for the birth?
A Certainly in every labour a midwife will carry out routine checks, such as listening to your baby's heartbeat and measuring your blood pressure. But beyond this hospitals vary in their approach to labour. Some expect staff to follow so many protocols that it considerably reduces your options; others are much more open to individual choices (see Hospital birth, page 24).

Q I do not think I will get the sort of birth I want at the hospital my doctor has sent me to. My first baby is due in three weeks. Is it too late to have a home birth?
A Why are you seeing a doctor and not a midwife? You are entitled to change your mind and be referred to a different hospital or a midwife unit, or to choose a home birth at any time. If your midwife feels a home birth is risky in your case, listen to the reasons. Making a decision means taking responsibility for the outcome, so be sure in your own mind what you want and take control.

Q What happens if a complication arises during the birth in a midwife unit?
A You should be aware that midwife units have no facilities for administering epidurals and no special-care baby unit. Should a complication arise during the birth, you will be moved to a consultant unit in a hospital, which is often close by.

Your birth plan

Most women formulate a general idea about the sort of birth they want by reading books, talking to their partner or other parents, and listening to advice offered by their midwife. Regardless of what other people think, you have to decide what you see as the advantages and disadvantages of the different approaches to labour and birth.

Writing a birth plan

By setting down a birth plan on paper you can think about what is important to you and your partner. A written birth plan acts as a communication tool between you and your midwife and helps to set the 'tone' of the sort of labour and birth you are hoping for. It can make you more realistic about what you are likely to experience, and may even prompt you to change your mind about where you want to give birth. For example, it may be easier to achieve a natural birth at home. Staff in a hospital may see a need to use technology – speeding up labour with drugs for instance – whereas a midwife at a home birth may consider it unnecessary.

The best way of presenting a birth plan is in the form of a letter. This is far more personal than the various printed forms available and will give the midwife caring for you some idea of your personality. Put something of yourself into the plan, and explain what you and your partner feel is important and why.

Birth plan checklist

Here are 15 questions to ask yourself:

1 Do you want your birth partner(s) present throughout labour and birth or only during certain procedures?
2 Do you have special needs because of language, a disability, your religion or diet?
3 Do you prefer to be cared for by women?
4 Do you want to know the midwife who cares for you in labour?
5 Do you mind a student being present during labour and birth?
6 Do you want to be encouraged to move about during labour?
7 Have you considered all your options for pain relief (see Chapter 2)?
8 Do you want to avoid constant fetal monitoring, which would stop you moving about during labour? (See Monitoring the baby, page 74.)
9 What are your views on induced labour – do you want your waters broken only if necessary? (See Induced labour, page 72.)
10 Under what circumstances would you be prepared to have an episiotomy? (See Episiotomy and tearing, page 88.)
11 Do you want to deliver the placenta without intervention? (See Stage 3 of labour, page 78.)
12 Does your partner want to cut the cord?
13 Do you want to see the sex of your baby yourself rather than be told?
14 Do you want your baby delivered onto your abdomen?
15 Do you want to put your baby straight to the breast?

Your birth plan **Common questions**

Q Is it better to lie down or to adopt an upright position during labour and birth?
A Generally speaking, lying down prolongs labour. Upright positions work with gravity; they tend to speed up labour and help to move your baby further down the birth canal. (See also pages 68 and 77.)

Q What methods might be used to induce or speed up labour?
A A midwife may break your waters to speed up labour, although this might make it more intense and painful. If this fails, a hormone drip may be needed (see page 72). This also shortens labour, but your baby may become distressed so you will be constantly monitored and your movement may be restricted. Some labours are naturally longer than others. Beware of speeding it up unnecessarily.

Q Is it better to tear than to be given an episiotomy?
A In most cases, it appears to be better to tear than to be cut. Tears do not always go through the muscle, and may just involve the skin, whereas a cut goes through both skin and muscle. It also appears that tears heal better and are more comfortable than a cut. If you tear, you might not even need stitches – a small tear will heal just as well as long as it is left alone but kept clean to reduce any risk of infection.

Q Can I deliver the placenta naturally?
A You can list this as a preference on your birth plan, and there is no reason why you cannot deliver the placenta naturally if you have had a normal birth with no risk of bleeding. Leaving the umbilical cord to pulsate may mean up to an hour's wait for the placenta, but the baby gets extra blood and a gentler transition into breathing. In all other situations – for example, if there is a risk of bleeding, you had a drip to induce labour, an epidural or pethidine, and in the case of a forceps or ventouse delivery – the midwife will advise you to have an injection to speed up delivery of the placenta.

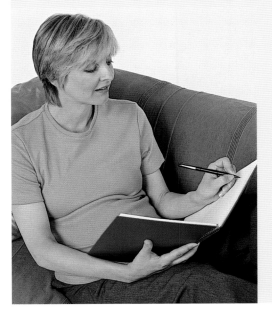

Left: Writing a birth plan is an effective way of communicating your wishes to the midwife.

Hospital birth

For many women, having a baby is their first experience of being in a hospital. Suddenly finding yourself in an unfamiliar environment, surrounded by strange equipment can be very unnerving. Ideally, part of your antenatal care should include a tour of the maternity unit where your baby will be born. You will have the opportunity to see the equipment and familiarize yourself with the environment.

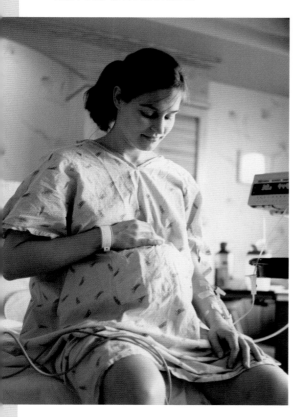

Most hospitals provide tours of the labour suite, often at evenings or weekends so that partners can attend. Such a visit is worth making so that you can learn what facilities are available and the various instruments that may be used. You can also take this opportunity to find out whether your hospital is geared more towards a 'high-tech' or a 'low-tech' birth, or somewhere in between (see page 28). If you do not discover this until you are in labour, you will be too preoccupied to ask questions that could help reduce any anxiety.

Hospital equipment

Most hospital rooms are equipped with a range of devices in addition to the bed, which is usually in the centre of the room so that people can move around it. The equipment will include the following items.

• **A cardiotocograph (CTG)** – to monitor your baby's heartbeat and your contractions.

• **A Doppler** – a handheld device for listening to your baby's heartbeat.

• **Gas and air (Entonox)** – which may be piped through a tube in the wall of the room or in a canister, and has a mouthpiece or facemask attached to it.

• **A sphygmomanometer** – to measure your blood pressure, which will be checked at various times throughout labour.

Left: Women who feel reassured by proximity to birth technology may opt for a hospital birth.

What do your notes mean?

If there is anything in your notes that you do not understand, it is better to ask than to go home and worry. Here are some common phrases and abbreviations.

Your details	**G:** Gravida, or number of pregnancies • **P, or Para:** Refers to the number of live births. For example G3P2 means third pregnancy, two live births **LB/SB:** Live birth/Stillbirth • **TCA 3/7 (4/52):** To come again in three days (or four weeks) • **Brim:** The inlet or upper rim of your pelvis • **Fundus:** The top of your uterus, which rises as your baby grows and descends a little when your baby's head engages (see Your baby's position, below) **BP:** Blood pressure • **PET:** Pre-eclampsia (pre-eclamptic toxaemia) **US, or USS:** Ultrasound scan.
Urine	**NAD:** Nothing abnormal detected • **Alb/Tr Prot+ (or ++):** Albumin/Trace of protein. Tr indicates a tiny amount of protein while three plus signs indicate a significant amount. This could signify the start of pre-eclampsia **0 Gluc:** No glucose found in the urine. Two plus signs or more would be considered high.
Blood	**Bloods:** Blood tests done • **FBC:** Full blood count • **Hb:** Haemoglobin count • **Fe:** Iron tablets. The prescription name may be recorded • **WR:** Syphilis test (Wasserman reaction). Alternatives are VDRL/TPHA (venereal disease research laboratory/Treponema pallidum haemagglutination) and FTA-Abs (fluorescent treponemal antibody absent).
Your baby's health	**FMF/FMNF:** Fetal movements felt/Fetal movements not felt • **FHH/FHNH:** Fetal heart heard/Fetal heart not heard. The heart rate (usually between 120 and 160 beats per minute) may be recorded • **FHHR:** Fetal heart heard regularly.
Your baby's position	**LOA/ROA:** Left occipito anterior/Right occipito anterior. The presenting part of your baby – the part nearest to the cervix and likely to emerge first **LOP/ROP** Left occipito posterior/Right occipito posterior. See above **Vx or Ceph:** Vertex or cephalic, meaning 'head down' • **Br/Tr:** Breech (bottom down)/Transverse (lying across the uterus) • **Eng, or E:** Engaged. This refers to how far down your baby's head is in your pelvis. When recorded in fifths it refers to the proportion of your baby's head above the brim of your pelvis. So 2/5 means the head is fully engaged, ready for the birth, while 4/5 means it has started to engage • **N/Eng, or NE:** Not engaged.

Hospital birth
Who's who on the ward

With a low-risk pregnancy, there is no need for anyone other than a midwife to care for you. This also applies to labour. The midwife is the expert in 'normality' and will only involve a doctor if there are any complications or concerns. She will also care for the well-being of you and your baby in the days following the birth.

There are occasions when you will meet other staff on the labour ward. They include the following people.

• **An obstetrician** This is a doctor who specializes in the care of women who have complications during pregnancy, labour or in the immediate post-natal period.

• **An anaesthetist** This is a doctor who specializes in anaesthetics and is responsible for putting an epidural in position. If you need to go to an operating theatre, an anaesthetist will be present, not only to provide an epidural or general anaesthetic, but also to assist if excessive bleeding occurs and to monitor your vital signs.

• **A paediatrician** This is a doctor who specializes in babies and child health, and who may check your baby after the birth. A paediatrician is present at instrumental deliveries or if any problem is anticipated with a baby, for example, premature labour.

• **Students** Looking after women in labour is obviously an essential part of some students'

Six questions to ask about the labour ward

There are six main things you need to know about the labour ward.

1 How many birth partners can you have?
2 What use can you make of the furniture in the room you will occupy during labour? (Does the bed have multiple positions? Is there room for a large beanbag or rocking chair? Can you bring your own birthing ball?)
3 What is the hospital's rate of births by caesarean section compared to normal vaginal births?
4 What are the visiting arrangements? (Are visiting times restricted? Are other children, such as siblings, allowed on the ward? What facilities are there for car-parking?)
5 Is there a birthing pool? What percentage of the midwives attend water births?
6 How do you gain access to the maternity unit at night? (Hospital security procedures may mean that the door you would normally use is locked.)

training, but you should always be asked whether you want them to be present and you have a right to refuse.

• **Other staff** There will be a number of other people on the labour ward, such as health-care assistants, porters and theatre staff.

True
story

A hospital's midwife unit

'The day before my due date, I had a pedicure and my hair cut. At about 5pm I went to the bathroom and noticed that I'd had a "show". Later that evening, I was in the bathroom again and had an irresistible urge to clean the shower. I'd never believed in the nesting instinct, but it obviously happens!

'At 8.30pm I finished a long phone call and realized, as I rang off, that my back was starting to hurt. Within the next 30 minutes the pain got stronger and, despite all my efforts to prevent a backache labour, the pain did seem to be all in my back.

'An hour later I called Tahir's parents, who live an hour away, to drive us to the hospital because Tahir can't drive. While we waited, I walked around and got down on all fours, which seemed to help.

'By 11pm Tahir's parents still hadn't arrived and the pain was unbearable. He phoned the hospital to ask if they could send an ambulance. Luckily, a few minutes later his mum and dad turned up. I was very relieved, as I was starting to think that I'd have my baby in the hallway!

'I was booked into the midwife-led unit of the local hospital, and as soon as we arrived, just after midnight, I could feel the peace and tranquillity taking over. The midwife examined me and said I was 7 cm (3 in) dilated, and that I was making great progress. Although I was still panicking about having a long backache labour, I trusted her judgement. She left us alone and I walked around and around. Tahir massaged my back when it all got too much.

'At 2.20am the midwife said I was ready to push, but I had absolutely no urge to do so. She asked me to hand over the gas and air mask, which I'd been getting quite attached to, and I started spontaneously pushing. After half an hour, she told me my baby had passed meconium, which I knew could be a sign of distress. This was all the motivation I needed. With two more pushes Delphine was born, at 2.53am. She was put straight to my breast and I felt a wonderful sense of achievement. I was euphoric that I'd managed an active, natural birth.'

Frederika, mother of Delphine

Hospital birth
High-tech and low-tech

A high-tech birth may involve a hormone drip to control contractions, a fetal monitor to record the baby's heartbeat, and an epidural to numb the pain. A low-tech approach involves no active intervention as long as you and your baby are fine. You could cope with contractions using relaxation and breathing techniques, and pain relief is on hand if you need it.

Most hospitals adopt a mixed approach: basically low-tech but with guidelines regarding, for example, when a drip should be used to speed up labour or how long you should push before needing an assisted birth.

However, ultimately, it is for you to decide, in discussion with your midwife, when intervention is appropriate.

Levels of intervention

If this is your first baby, you may not necessarily know the level of intervention you would prefer (assuming that there are no complications). The questionnaire may help (see box). The more 'No' answers that you give then the more likely you are to be reassured by birth technology. The more 'Yes' answers, the more likely you are to prefer a natural approach. Staff in large hospitals may be more geared to using technology than those in small hospitals or health-care units. Home births are least likely to involve intervention in labour (see page 30).

Ten questions to **ask yourself**

Reply as honestly as possible to each question.

1 Do you mind the idea of being wired to machinery during labour?
2 Do you empathize with women who choose to give birth at home?
3 Would you prefer to move around and choose comfortable positions?
4 Do you believe that labour can be a natural event for most women?
5 Will you feel confident if your baby's heartbeat is not monitored throughout labour, just in case anything goes wrong?
6 Do you believe that relaxing in familiar surroundings can make labour easier?
7 Do you have any doubts that doctors and midwives always know what is best for you?
8 Would you prefer to have no intervention as long as your baby is all right?
9 Would you prefer to avoid drugs if possible?
10 Do you disagree with women who want whatever drugs are available, as long as they do not have to feel anything?

Hospital birth **Common questions**

Q Will intervention be inevitable in all hospital births?

A Intervention is a matter of judgement and depends partly on the philosophy of the hospital and its staff. Some hospitals advocate intervention before any problem occurs, in the hope of preventing a difficult or dangerous situation arising. Other hospitals favour watching carefully but not intervening until there is a problem, in the belief that intervention can itself cause problems. The technology is there for them to use if a complication occurs, but there is no evidence to suggest that it makes birth any safer if everything is proceeding normally.

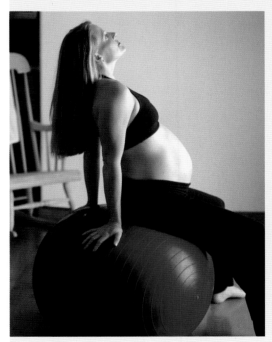

Above: Ask your hospital about any equipment, such as birthing balls, that they may be able to provide.

Q Do I have to lie down throughout labour?

A Even in a high-tech birth, you do not have to lie down, although many women do end up on the bed. It will be possible to raise your bed, either manually or electronically, and it will have stirrups in case of a forceps or a ventouse delivery. Many beds can be converted into birthing chairs by removing the end and putting the head upright. Some hospitals offer the option of having a mattress on the floor.

Q What other birthing aids might be available to me at the hospital?

A There are a number of items that you need to ask about in advance, as they will probably be stored elsewhere in the hospital or are things that you yourself should provide. Birthing aids include a large beanbag, birthing ball or rocking chair, for encouraging a more active birth, and essential oils or CDs to create a relaxing atmosphere. The use of birthing pools is becoming more widespread, and many maternity units have more than one delivery unit with a pool.

Q How long will I stay in hospital?

A This depends on the sort of birth and how well you and your baby are. In most hospitals you can leave from the labour ward or stay for a few days after your baby's birth. Even with a first baby, mothers go home within hours, and most leave within a day or two. Your midwife will visit you at home to check on your well-being and support you with feeding and baby care. (See also Length of stay, page 106.)

Home birth

The biggest advantage to having your baby at home is being in a familiar, comfortable environment with none of the elements of uncertainty and fear that can inhibit labour in a hospital. You have the freedom to move around as you wish, and to have as many people with you as you choose – or you may just prefer to have the privacy, knowing that members of staff are not going to walk through the door. Women who have a home birth are more likely to feel in control and relaxed than those who give birth in a hospital.

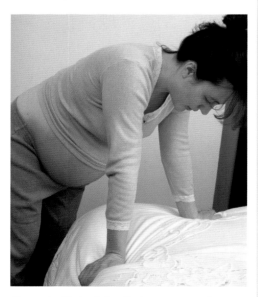

Above: Just being in familiar home surroundings can make women more relaxed during labour.

Preparing for a home birth

If you choose to have your baby at home, your midwife will generally bring all the delivery equipment to your house at around 37 weeks and leave it there. It will include gas and air, and baby resuscitation equipment, all of which she will talk through with you.

Six things to check for a home birth

There is little preparation involved in a home birth, but there are a few things you can do to make things easier.

1 Have your midwife's telephone number to hand – it is a good idea to have her mobile number as well as that of the community midwife office.

2 Walk around your house to see how you can use the furniture during labour. Ideally you want to remain upright and walking around.

3 Have an adjustable desk lamp or torch to hand so that the midwife can examine your perineum after the birth to see if you need any stitches.

4 Arrange for someone to take care of your other children, if any, in case you need to go to hospital.

5 Find some plastic sheeting, such as a ground sheet or old shower curtain, to protect your mattress or carpet. Old sheets or towels can also be useful.

6 Pack a bag for the hospital, just in case.

Home birth **Common questions**

Q How safe is a home birth?

A Evidence shows that, in a straightforward pregnancy, it is not safer to have your baby in hospital. Home is just as safe, and many would argue safer, because of the one-to-one care that you will receive from your midwife. With a hospital birth you are more likely to end up with interventions, and you have a greater risk of infection. Even if you are taken to hospital during labour, you are still less likely to end up with a caesarean section than someone booked for a hospital birth.

Q Under what circumstances would a home birth not be recommended?

A You can opt for a home birth in almost any circumstances – if you are over 35, are of small stature, are having your first baby, or have a history of problems in pregnancy or labour – as long as this pregnancy progresses without complications. A home birth is not recommended if you have pre-eclampsia (see page 13), or if your baby's growth in the uterus has been restricted (pre-eclampsia is a major cause), or if you have certain medical conditions, such as heart trouble, that could be exacerbated by labour.

Q What will actually happen during a home birth?

A Your midwife will come to your house and, once labour is established, will stay with you until the baby is born. You are free to do as you please in order to make yourself comfortable – eat and drink, walk about the room, meditate or take a bath – with your midwife observing you, checking your blood pressure and your baby's heartbeat. After the birth, she will clear up. She will then check over you and your baby, write her notes and, when you are settled and everything is tidy, leave a telephone number in case you need her. She will make routine visits to check you and your baby over the next few days, as you feel necessary.

Q What happens if there is a complication?

A Midwives are trained and equipped to deal with any emergencies that may arise. However, if there are signs that all is not well during labour, your midwife may advise you to go to hospital. You should discuss on what grounds she will do this beforehand. They will probably include your baby showing signs of distress during labour, including opening his bowels; very slow progress of labour; any bleeding during labour; high blood pressure; and signs of infection.

Home birth
Pain relief

Choosing to have a home birth makes a huge difference to a woman's ability to cope with the contractions. Because of this, and the one-to-one care that they get from the midwife, many women find that they do not need pain relief when they have a home birth. Most women use what is around them – they walk about, listen to music, eat and drink and generally stay relaxed, which is the secret of staying in control of your labour.

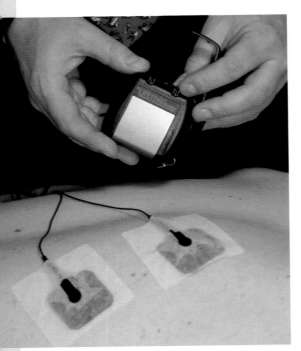

Above: A TENS machine, which encourages the release of endorphins, can be used in a home birth.

Types of pain relief

The reality is that many women are so relaxed to be going through labour and birth in the familiar surroundings of their own home that they don't need any pain relief at all. If pain relief is required, there is a wide range of effective natural and medical options suitable for use in a non-hospital setting. Many women find a soak in a warm (but not hot) bath to be a great source of natural pain relief, while others may like to be massaged or to have hot towels applied to the lower back by their birth partner. An epidural is always administered by an anaesthetist and is therefore not appropriate for a home birth, but other forms of pain-relief technology are available.

• You can use a **transcutaneous electrical nerve stimulation** (TENS) machine, which works by blocking the pain impulses and encouraging your body to produce natural painkillers (endorphins). Ask your midwife if she can bring one with her or whether you should hire one.

• You can use **gas and air** (Entonox) to take the edge off the pain. Your midwife will bring some canisters to your home and you can breathe the mixture of nitrous oxide and oxygen through a mouthpiece or facemask.

• Some doctors will prescribe **meptazinol or pethidine** for the midwife to give you. However, some midwives are reluctant to use these mood-altering drugs at home because they can make the baby drowsy and the baby will require close monitoring (see Medical pain relief, page 52, for more information about these treatments).

True story

A typical home birth

'I decided on a home birth, after months of deliberation. I was not keen at first, as I thought it was riskier than in hospital. But I changed my mind because I needed my parents to mind Abby and they lived more than half an hour away, which could be tricky if I needed to go to hospital in the middle of the night.

'The first sign was a popping feeling, and the realization that I was a bit "damp". Five minutes later I had a mild contraction. My husband Tony begged me to ring the midwife and, after about 45 minutes, I agreed. I had a contraction while I was on the phone to her, but as I could talk through it I did not think I was in proper labour. Julie, my midwife, said she would come and check me over anyway. I was a bit despondent, assuming that I had a long night and, possibly, day ahead.

'But that was not the case. Within ten minutes of speaking to Julie, I had a long, painful contraction. I immediately regretted not ringing her earlier, and I started to panic about how we would cope if she did not make it in time. Tony inflated the air mattress we had bought especially for the lounge and then just paced the floor.

'Julie turned up when the contractions were only three minutes apart and very long. I continued to labour away while Tony and Julie chatted. Suddenly I had the urge to push. Julie examined me, threw her keys at Tony, instructing him to get her bag out of her car, and then told him to phone the hospital for her. She told them that the baby would arrive within ten minutes and that the other midwife would be too late.

'I made a lot of noise during the pushing phase as I had not had time for any pain relief. Part of me was glad it was nearly over, but I was also thinking how much it was going to hurt. The noise woke Abby, who came downstairs to see what was going on. Having worried before that this could happen, I had tried to prepare her by talking about it, as well as watching real-life births on the television with her. She was standing slightly behind my shoulders, clinging onto her daddy. As baby Charlotte was born, I turned to look at Abby and she had a huge grin on her face. Shortly afterwards, my parents arrived.

'Giving birth at home was really amazing. I would not hesitate next time, but maybe Tony should brush up on his midwifery skills just in case it is even quicker!'
Donna, mother of Abby and Charlotte

WATER BIRTH

Easing your baby's passage into the world

A birthing pool can provide natural pain relief and a soothing environment for mother and baby, but it is not suitable for use in all births.

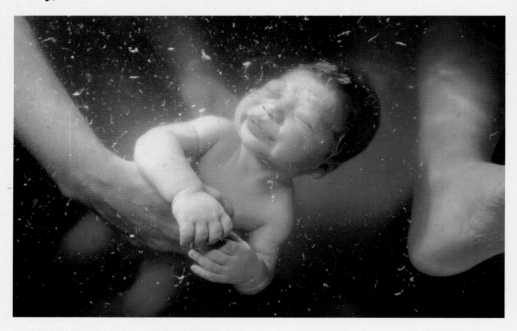

Above: A baby born under water in a birthing pool will not try to breathe until brought to the surface.

'I had a water birth and the minute I got into the pool the difference was amazing. I had been feeling the contractions across my lower back but the warm water relieved this and I was able to relax.'
Paulette, mother of Grace

The idea of a water birth was originally explored by Russian Igor Tcharkovsky in the early 1970s. He discovered that newborns have a so-called 'dive reflex': like dolphins, they start trying to breathe only when they are brought to the surface of the water and come into contact with the air. Therefore, a baby can stay under water safely for the first few seconds of its life.

Whether or not a water birth is a suitable option for you depends on your type of

Five reasons for considering a **water birth**

There are several advantages to a water birth.

1 Water encourages relaxation, greater mobility and calmness, all of which help you to cope better with pain. It also supports your body, making it easier to change position and move around the pool.
2 Water can help prevent or lessen the risk of tears, by helping the vagina to stretch and soften. This will ease your baby's passage into the world.
3 It can speed up labour by stimulating better hormone secretion. Immersion in water stimulates the production of oxytocin, which can bring about more powerful contractions and therefore faster dilation of the cervix.
4 Water reinforces a feeling of privacy and personal space. Midwives often interfere less if you are in a birthing pool, although they do periodically check your blood pressure and your baby's heart rate.
5 The transition from the sanctuary of the amniotic sac to the dramatically different outside world is smoother and easier for a newborn if she first finds herself in a familiar watery environment.

second stage of labour, it should be 37°C. Birthing pools vary in size, but they are usually large enough for one person to move around freely. The water usually reaches just above your bump when you are sitting or squatting inside it. You can use the buoyancy of the water to change position whenever you feel the need.

Some women opt to use the pool during the first stage of labour (when the contractions are working to dilate the cervix) and then, once they are fully dilated, get out for the birth. If you have had a long, tiring labour, you may feel it is easier to give birth out of the pool because gravity will assist you. However, if you choose to deliver in the water, your baby will be gently guided to the surface by you, your birth partner or your midwife.

If you would like a water birth, consider hiring a birthing pool, either to use at home or to take to the maternity unit if it does not have one already. Remember that hospital birthing facilities are subject to availability and work on a 'first come, first served' basis.

The basic criteria for having a water birth are as follows:

• You have to be at least 37 weeks pregnant. Premature babies may still be underdeveloped and should not be born in a pool.
• Your baby should be lying head down because this is the easiest and safest position for her descent into the water.
• If you are carrying twins, you would normally be advised against a water birth because of the increased risk of complications.
• You will not be able to use the pool if you have had an epidural or pethidine (these pain relief options are not available for a water birth). You can, however, use gas and air.

pregnancy. In medical terms, you need a low-risk pregnancy with no obstetric complications. A flexible attitude is important: every birth is unpredictable, and if you do not appear to be coping well with the pain, or your labour is not progressing as expected, you may want to get out of the pool. Assuming all is well, you will be able to get back into the pool later on.

The water in the pool should be at a temperature that you find comfortable. In the

Birth partners

The greatest influence on your ability to cope during labour is the support that you receive. This will come not only from your midwife, but also from the person, or persons, you choose to have with you at the birth. You need to feel confident that they will be able to give you emotional support and practical care. Research has shown that women who have continual support during labour are more confident about motherhood, more likely to have a positive experience of birth, and less likely to suffer from depression at six weeks after the birth.

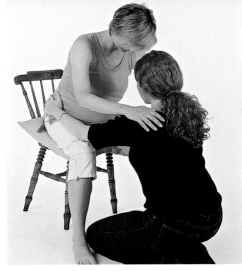

Above: Some women choose a female friend or relative as their birth partner.

Although most fathers want to be at the birth, this is not right for every couple. The most important thing is to have good support in labour, regardless of who provides it. In some cultures, fathers are discouraged from attending a birth and two female relatives attend instead. You must trust the people you choose to stay with you and be honest about what you expect from them during your labour – but essentially they should want to be there.

True story

'Albert has supported me through each of my labours by encouraging me whenever I began to doubt my ability to continue. Sophie was eight weeks premature, so I was very scared about the outcome. Albert was really supportive and stayed by my side throughout, talking and breathing with me. At one point I nearly broke his thumb – which was weakened from a rugby injury – I was twisting and squeezing it so hard!

'Sophie's birth was particularly poignant as she was our first baby as a married couple. When she had to go straight into special care, Albert was strong for both of us. There was no one else I would have wanted to share the magic and joys of childbirth with. I felt that he should be there, especially as each of our children is just as much his as mine: to shut him out would not have been right.'
Sarah, mother of Jack, Alex and Sophie

Birth partners **Common questions**

Q How many birth partners can I have?
A Most maternity units are happy for two people to be with you during labour because research shows that continual support benefits mothers in a number of ways, such as feeling more in control of labour and more positive about the birth experience. Consider who would be best to provide this support. It may be your partner, a friend, a sister or your mother. Women who have had children before will not worry about seeing you in pain and are more able to reassure you that everything is completely normal.

Q My husband wants so much to be at the birth, but he is anxious about how he will cope with it all. How can I encourage him?
A Many men have fears about birth, the most common being concerns about seeing their partner in pain and not being able to relieve them of it. Persuade your husband to attend antenatal classes with you. The opportunity to talk with other men in the group and to discover that he is not alone in his fears might make him more confident about being present at the birth.

Q My husband refuses to be my birth partner. I feel rejected and worried about coping alone. How can I persuade him to change his mind?
A Some men simply do not want to witness labour and birth, and you should not regard this attitude as a betrayal. Relationships work in different ways, and there is more to being a good husband or father than attending the birth. You will not be alone when your baby is born. Your midwife will provide help and companionship as part of her duties. Why not consider choosing a close relative or girlfriend to be your birth partner? She can attend antenatal classes with you and share your experience in a way that complements your husband's involvement. If your husband feels that there is no pressure, you may find that his feelings change and he wants to be more actively involved, perhaps staying for the early part of your labour. You might even end up with two birth partners working together!

'We decided at the outset that Stephen would not be with me for the birth, as he is not good in stressful situations. We chose instead a close female friend, who had also had a baby, and my mother. On the day, they knew what to do and were aware of the emotions women go through in labour. Stephen came under a lot of pressure, but it was a decision we made together and we would do the same again.'
Pamela, mother of Beth

Birth partners
Their role

Your birth partner will feel more confident in his role if you involve him early on in your pregnancy. A basic understanding of the process of labour will help to remove some of the anxiety. It is essential that your birth partner is there to help you cope with contractions. Above all he needs to listen to you and provide encouragement and emotional support.

How your birth partner can help

The following list provides a number of ways in which your birth partner can help you to stay relaxed during labour. He or she can:

- Provide you with drinks and snacks while you are at home waiting for your contractions to get close enough together, reminding you to eat and drink.

- Give you a supporting arm if you want to take a walk and need reassurance.

- Encourage you to keep moving around, change positions and keep off the bed.

- Offer verbal encouragement and reassurance about how well you are doing.

- Help you to establish a pattern of breathing during your contractions.

- Talk to your midwife about aspects of your labour or birth plan if you do not feel up to it.

- Keep you cool by applying a cold flannel to your forehead or neck.

- Massage your back and shoulders, if this is what you want.

- Support you if you want to sit up or lean forward during the second phase of labour.

- Encourage you during the last stage of labour by keeping you informed about the progress of your baby's head.

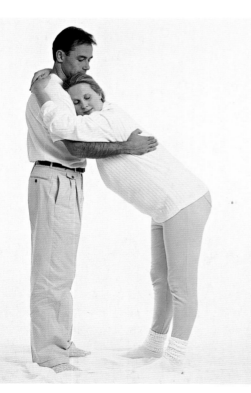

Above: Your birth partner can support you both physically and emotionally.

Birth partners **Common questions**

Q What is a doula?

A The word 'doula' comes from a Greek word meaning 'a woman care-giver'. It has come to mean a woman, experienced in childbirth, who provides emotional and practical support to another woman during and after birth. She is well informed, understands the physiology of birth, and can help you and your partner make informed decisions on the choices that are available to you. Her aim is to make the experience of labour and childbirth more positive. During labour, she will help you with breathing and relaxation and encourage you to change positions as your labour progresses.

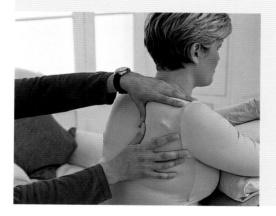

Q My teenage daughter from my husband's first marriage wants to be present at the birth. We have asked my mother-in-law to look after our 3-year-old son, who adores his Gran. How can I prepare my stepdaughter for the birth and ensure my son does not feel left out?

A Your daughter might like to look at books or a video with you, and she should be aware of the practicalities of birth. Tell her that she can leave at any time if she wishes and explain the circumstances in which you might not be comfortable with her present. Make sure that your midwife knows that she will be there, so that she will feel welcome. If a day spent with undivided attention is a treat for your son, he is unlikely to feel left out. He may not be at the birth but he can still be part of the celebrations: your mother-in-law could help him to decorate a card for the baby. Consider a home birth – make it a family celebration, with everyone having the option of being there!

Left: An experienced doula will help you with your posture, breathing and relaxation during labour.

Single mothers

As a single mother you are entitled to have a birth partner – perhaps your mother, a friend or a family member. Choose someone you can rely on and with whom you feel comfortable. This person could also attend antenatal classes with you. There may be classes aimed at single women in your area – ask your midwife.

Looking after your baby 24 hours a day can be lonely, particularly if you are tired and he is crying. Do not be too proud to accept help from family members or friends – it does not mean that you are not coping. If you have no one to help you, tell your doctor or midwife, who can recommend sources of support.

Are you ready?

As the birth approaches, make sure you have everything ready and to hand. Once you go into labour, you must go to the maternity unit. It is worth calling first to let them know you are on your way. If you have had a tour of the unit, you will know where to go when you arrive.

Phone numbers

Know who to ring when you go into labour. You should have the phone number of the maternity unit in your antenatal notes, as well as any other important phone numbers, such as your community midwife or ambulance control. It is always useful to have a list of other phone numbers to hand – not only your partner's mobile number, but also the numbers of local taxi firms and people you will want to call with your news after the birth.

Getting there

Make sure that you and your partner know how to get to the maternity unit. You would be amazed at the number of people who get lost on the way! You could even practise driving the route in the rush hour, just to see how long it takes. Remember that, with a first baby, even if you get stuck in traffic, you will probably still have time to spare. Make sure that you can find the correct entrance, especially at night when the main doors to the hospital or maternity unit may be locked.

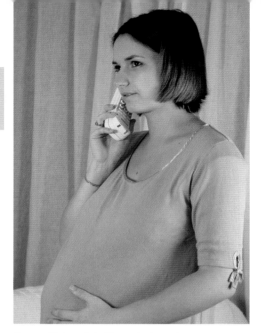

Above: Make a list of important numbers, so you can reach your midwife and other contacts quickly.

Are you ready?
Common questions

Q What should I pack for the hospital? I have no idea how long I will be there for, or what my body will be like after the birth.
A It is useful to pack two bags: one for the labour ward and one for the post-natal ward (see box). Even if you are planning to have your baby at home, pack a bag for the labour ward in case you need to be transferred to hospital during your labour. Do not be too ambitious and think that you will be able to wear your normal clothes after the birth – it will be a few weeks before you can get into your pre-maternity wear. Keep your packing to a minimum and get your partner to take home any soiled clothing that you wore to the hospital or during labour, and to bring you fresh replacements for when you go home.

What shall I pack?

Your hospital will provide a list of things to bring, and here are some additional suggestions. It is easier to pack things into two separate bags.

Labour ward bag

- Comfortable clothes to wear during labour, such as an extra large T-shirt or nightdress
- Socks and slippers
- Dressing gown
- Three pairs of large disposable knickers (for when your waters break and also immediately after the birth, when your blood loss will be quite heavy)
- Clean nightdress for after the birth
- A sponge or flannel for keeping you cool during labour
- Massage oils if you have decided to use them
- Toiletries, including mild soap, toothbrush and toothpaste, hairbrush and towel
- Sanitary towels (maternity pads or night-time sanitary towels)
- Cartons of fruit juice and some high-energy snacks (such as dried fruits)
- Birth plan
- Camera
- Hot-water bottle for easing any backache
- Hand mirror – so that you can see your baby's head emerging, especially useful when you feel you are not making any progress
- Battery-operated cassette recorder or radio (note that electronic items may not be allowed on the ward) and a selection of music that you can focus on through your contractions. Check to see what is provided
- Change for the telephone (you may not be allowed to use a mobile phone in hospital), address book and important telephone numbers
- For your baby: three stretch suits, three vests, nappies, cotton wool, a hat

Post-natal ward bag

- Nightdress – front-opening if you intend to breastfeed
- Several pairs of knickers
- Nursing bra
- A few breast pads
- Good-quality nipple cream
- Sanitary towels (heavy-duty)
- Something to read – if you get the time!

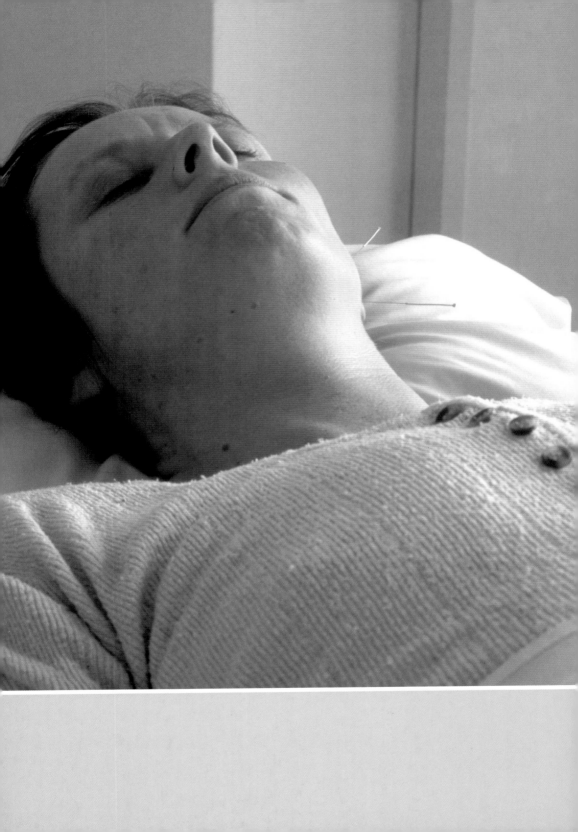

2

handling pain

Natural pain relief

You can never judge in advance what pain relief, if any, you will want during labour. Keep an open mind about the different options because many factors influence labour, including the baby's position (see page 56), whether or not labour is induced (see page 72) and even the shape of the pelvis. While various types of medical pain relief are on offer for a hospital or home birth (see pages 32 and 52), many women are now using alternative methods rather than automatically considering medication.

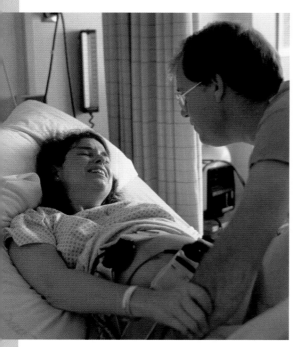

The natural way

Giving birth is a natural process and, unless there are complications, the vast majority of women are capable of giving birth without medication. There are many ways in which you can deal with your contractions that do not involve using drugs. The most important thing for you and your partner is to accept that you cannot banish the pain, only find ways of coping with it.

One means of handling pain is to try to keep active, staying on your feet and moving around. Being upright can reduce the length of your labour and increase your ability to cope with contractions. Maintaining a realistic and positive approach, and being able to relax, also raises your pain threshold.

If possible, try to view the pain you are experiencing positively – remind yourself that each contraction is bringing the birth of your baby closer. Self-help methods of pain relief can help you feel more relaxed and in control. Such an approach is all about empowerment and enabling yourself to play an active role in your baby's birth.

Most of the techniques for natural pain relief (see chart, page 46) are based on relaxation. Unfortunately, fear has a negative effect on the body during labour, slowing down contractions, tensing muscles and increasing pain. Alternative forms of pain relief put a great deal of emphasis on relaxation with the release of endorphins, the body's natural painkillers.

Left: Your birth partner can offer reassurance and encouragement as you cope with pain.

True story

Birth without pain relief

'During my second pregnancy, I was very apprehensive and scared about going into labour. Memories of the birth of my son, Austin (which involved gas, pethidine, intense pain, lots of yelling and very tensed-up muscles), were still at the front of my mind and I'd decided that an epidural was my best option this time round.

'Not long after reading an article on hypnotherapy, I was talking to one of my sister's friends about her experience of it, and I thought, "Wow! That sounds interesting." I'd done a couple of yoga courses, so I knew about breathing and how it can relax your body. I decided to contact a local practitioner and sign up for a course.

'At the first session, our small group of couples was told that with hypnotherapy techniques, a pain- and drug-free labour was possible, and that this has been a reality for many women around the world. To reinforce this, we were shown a video of women in labour peacefully using the techniques. In subsequent sessions, we were introduced to breathing techniques, affirmations and visualization exercises that could be used during labour.

'I can't tell you what a huge difference it made. Compared to my first labour, this one was half as long, and totally drug-free. The seven hours seemed like just a few, and I felt so much better after the birth. I was able to focus on relaxing my body during labour and only experienced intense pressure in the last half hour. I kept thinking that the more I could relax, the more effective each contraction would be and the sooner my baby would arrive.

'Also, this time Liam played a pivotal role. He kept me focused on my breathing and really directed my thoughts towards staying totally relaxed and using the visualizations that we'd practised together. There was no comparison to my first birth – at the antenatal classes they had focused on how painful it was going to be, but didn't really give any strategies for dealing with it. In my first labour, Liam admitted that he felt totally useless – all he could do was just give me ice chips. This time round I think he felt he was really part of it.

'The midwives were fantastic, but I didn't rely on them as much. They were all amazed by the effects of hypnotherapy and even my consultant wanted to know more!'

Sharon, mother of Austin and Georgia

Natural pain relief
The options

	What to do	How it works
Relaxation	Learn how to release the tension in your muscles by breathing (see page 58). Relax your face, which will automatically relax your other muscles. Focus on some mental image, or listen to a special piece of music, to distract you from the contractions and to help you to relax through them.	Relaxing tense muscles encourages the body to produce endorphins, the natural painkillers.
Water	Relax in a warm bath. If you have backache, take a shower and aim the showerhead at the base of your spine. Placing a hot-water bottle or towels soaked in warm water on your back may help, particularly if you have backache during labour.	The warmth relaxes the muscles, reducing tension and pain and helping your body to produce natural endorphins.
Massage and aromatherapy	You will be reliant on your birth partner for this. Research suggests that, just by visualizing your partner's hand massaging you, your body will release oxytocin, which helps the contractions to keep coming. Try putting a few drops of clary sage, jasmine or rose oil on a handkerchief to inhale during labour.	Massage is soothing and comforting, as well as relaxing tense muscles.
Transcutaneous electrical nerve stimulation (TENS)	A TENS machine consists of a small portable handset and sticky electrode pads that you attach to your back.	With every contraction, the machine releases small electrical impulses that block the pain and encourage the body to release endorphins.
Hypnotherapy	Courses are available in self-hypnosis and breathing techniques designed for labour and birth (see What is hypnotherapy? page 49).	Uses self-hypnosis, deep relaxation, visualization, anxiety management and breathing techniques to keep you feeling positive and in control.

Advantages	Disadvantages	Effectiveness
Safe for you and your baby. You can stay active. Even if you are having a vaginal examination, or waiting for an epidural or pethidine to take effect, it helps to know how to relax.	None.	Relaxation will help you cope with the pain.
Safe for you and your baby. Suitable both at home and in hospital. Water supports the weight of your body and you can change positions easily.	None.	These measures will help you cope with pain by making you more relaxed, so the experience of pain is reduced.
Safe for you and your baby. Can work well in any position. Can be used with other methods of pain relief.	You may not feel like being touched when it comes to labour. Some essential oils should not be used during pregnancy – check with an aromatherapist.	Massage can be effective in helping you cope – particularly with backache during labour.
Safe for you and your baby. Can be used at home or in hospital. You are in control of its use and movement is not restricted. Easily removed if it does not work.	May need to be hired from a major drugstore or baby-care shop (not all maternity units have a machine, or it might already be in use). Cannot be used in a birthing pool.	Reports vary. Some women find TENS inadequate. Others say they could not have managed without it. It may be most helpful during early labour.
Safe for you and your baby. Can be used at home or in hospital. You are in control. Movement is encouraged. No equipment is necessary.	Courses are not universally available and those that are accessible may be expensive.	Users of the techniques report less pain and stress, shorter labour, fewer complications and medical or surgical interventions, quicker recovery times and better bonding with their babies.

Natural pain relief
Complementary therapy

There are various complementary therapies that offer a combination of pain relief and relaxation, as well as stimulating the release of endorphins, which are the body's natural painkillers. If this approach is one of your options, be sure to consult a registered therapist.

True story

Giving birth with natural pain relief

'I had a wonderful pregnancy, which was a pleasant surprise. The day before my due date, at around midday, I started getting pains unlike any I had experienced before, but I put them down to Braxton Hicks. When my partner Neil came home, he suggested calling the hospital. The midwife said it sounded like early labour and told me to come in when I could no longer bear the pain.

'By early evening the pains were worse and coming five minutes apart. I waited as long as I could, and then we went to the hospital. We arrived at 8.45pm. The midwife checked me and called the doctor, as she thought my baby might be breech. Luckily the baby was head down and I was 3 cm (about 1¼ in) dilated. The next four hours were hard work. The contractions intensified and were more painful when I lay down or kept still, so I stayed upright, walking and rocking my pelvis. Neil was great, rubbing my back or not rubbing it, putting on my socks and then taking them off. At 2.30am, the midwife checked me and found that I was 7 cm (3 in) dilated. I was so relieved – my baby was on her way.

'I got into the birthing pool. As soon as my bump was immersed, I felt instant relief and totally relaxed. "In another three hours," said the midwife, "your baby will be here." But ten minutes later I had an uncontrollable urge to push. The midwives told me to follow my body, so I just went with it and pushed. Around 40 minutes later they told me the head was emerging and encouraged me to breathe the baby out. I felt in complete control and it was great. With one last push, Emilia was born. I looked down, and there she was in the water. The midwives asked if I wanted to lift her out, but I was afraid I might hurt her. They put her on my chest, and we sat in the pool for an hour. I felt so lucky to have had such a perfect labour. The feeling was so amazing and empowering that I cannot wait to do it again.'
Rachel, mother of Emilia

Complementary therapy **Common questions**

Q What is hypnotherapy?

A Hypnotherapy aims to help women release their anxiety about labour and giving birth or overcome fears created by previous traumatic birth experiences. This may be done through self-hypnosis, relaxation techniques and breathing exercises. Hypnotherapy does not mean that women undergo labour in a trance-like state, rather that they feel relaxed but in control and fully aware of what is going on. Courses are available and last about 12 hours, running over several weeks or a weekend. There are no prerequisites for taking a course, and it does not matter if you have doubts. With the help of hypnotherapy, even the most sceptical of participants can relax and release the fear and tension that make it difficult for muscles to work effectively during labour.

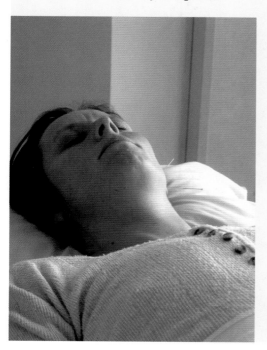

Q I have heard that acupuncture has been used to relieve pain during labour. What does this involve?

A The method is not dissimilar to using a TENS machine (see page 46). For women in labour, acupuncture points around the ear are often used, as this does not interfere with mobility. The needles in these points are then attached, via wires, to an electro-acupuncture machine, which you can control yourself. This stimulates the release of endorphins (the body's natural painkillers), helping to relieve pain, boost energy and aid relaxation. The effect takes about 20 minutes to build up, and your acupuncturist should stay with you while the machine is in use.

Q Is reflexology an alternative?

A Yes it is. Reflexology is a relaxing and calming therapy that involves massaging certain points on the feet, thereby stimulating the release of endorphins in the body. In addition, manipulation of the points on the ankle bone that are linked to the uterus and pelvis not only relieve the pain and anxiety of labour, but also help to regulate contractions. Your reflexologist will need to be available when you go into labour and should stay with you throughout.

Left: Techniques such as self-hypnosis and breathing exercices may help you to relax and manage pain.

Medical pain relief

Even if you are planning to give birth using natural pain relief (see page 46),you should also be aware of the different forms of medical relief. You will have no idea of your pain threshold until labour starts, and it may simply be too much for you to endure. You are not a failure if you opt for medical pain relief. The important thing is that you feel in control of your labour.

There are various options for medical pain relief, and each has its disadvantages as well as advantages. It therefore pays to consider them properly and rationally before going into labour. Gas and air (Entonox) makes some women feel nauseous or disorientated, while pethidine and other narcotic drugs can also affect the baby. If you are certain from the outset that you do want to use drugs to control the pain, then an epidural is the most effective method to choose.

Four reasons for choosing to have an **epidural**

Apart from its effectiveness, there are other advantages to having an epidural.

1 If you have high blood pressure, an epidural can help to lower it.
2 An epidural is useful for a long labour or if you feel unable to cope any longer.
3 The relief when the pain ceases makes you feel more in control and enables you to become more relaxed.
4 An epidural allows you to rest during a long labour and conserve energy, undisturbed by painful contractions.

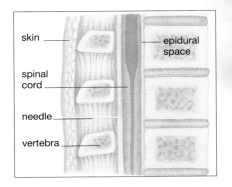

skin ——
spinal cord ——
needle ——
vertebra ——
—— epidural space

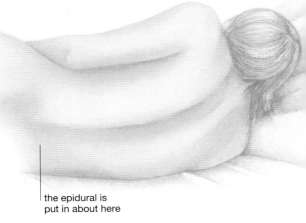

the epidural is put in about here

True
story

Giving birth with an epidural

'When I found out I was pregnant, I was thrilled to be having a baby, but the thought of giving birth actually made me cry. I honestly did not know how I was going to get through it. I wrote my birth plan and asked not to have an epidural or episiotomy because I had been watching births on TV and they looked scary.

'My fear abated a little as my pregnancy progressed and, when my waters broke, I calmly walked upstairs to the toilet and let John do the panicking. But, as the reality of it sank in, I started to shake, dreading the thought of the inevitable.

'My contractions started to get really painful once we arrived at the hospital. I asked for an epidural, despite the fact that I was scared of them. I realized I could not possibly tolerate any more pain. Unfortunately, the anaesthetist was elsewhere and I had to wait one long and painful hour with nothing but gas and air. However, the worst thing about the epidural was sitting still while it was administered. I did not even feel a scratch. In fact, the only thing I felt was the epidural liquid trickling down my spine and legs like liquid ice, which I actually found quite soothing. Once it kicked in, it was fantastic – utter relief!

'A few hours later I was ready to push. Still feeling no pain, I pushed for nearly two hours. I knew I was having a large baby, as at the 34-week scan he already weighed about 3.5 kg (7 lb 8 oz). A ventouse was tried but the apparatus kept slipping off the baby's head. They tried two or three times before suggesting forceps. I was reluctant because I was afraid that the baby would be scarred, but I didn't feel there was any option. This failed, too, and John and I looked at each other, both worrying that something was wrong.

'I was wheeled down to theatre for an emergency caesarean. I was crying at this point not only because I was scared for my baby, but also because I was terrified of being cut open. John disappeared to put on his scrubs. In the theatre, the doctor tried forceps one more time. I was in tears with fear and distress until my baby, Thomas, was born. Out he came, a little marked, but otherwise perfect.

'I am amazed at myself for what happened, but the thought of the epidural and birth was really ten times worse than the reality. I am so grateful to the midwives who helped with the birth. And I certainly will not be so scared next time!'
Kim, mother of Thomas

Medical pain relief
The options

	What happens	How it works	Advantages
Gas and air (Entonox)	Nitrous oxide and oxygen is inhaled through a mouthpiece or facemask.	Provides mild analgesia and relieves tension.	Safe for you and your baby. You control its use. No restrictions on movement. Can be used in a birthing pool. Clears quickly from the system. Helps to establish a breathing pattern for each contraction. Can be used with other methods of pain relief.
Pethidine or meptazinol	Narcotic drugs are injected into the buttock or thigh by a midwife. They take 20 minutes to have an effect and last for up to three hours.	Mood-altering, producing relaxation and drowsiness. Relieves tension and anxiety, which can both prolong labour.	Given by a midwife, so is readily available.
Epidural	Anaesthetic is introduced through a fine tube, inserted by an anaesthetist into the base of the spine. This can either be topped up by the midwife, as required, or given continuously through an infusion pump.	Numbs the area from the top of the bump downwards.	Can lower your blood pressure if it is very high. Will not affect the baby unless your blood pressure drops.
Spinal block	An anaesthetist injects anaesthetic into the fluid around the spinal cord to provide short-lasting but very effective pain relief and then removes the needle.	Numbs the area from the top of the bump downwards.	Can lower blood pressure if it is very high. Will not affect the baby, unless your blood pressure drops.

Disadvantages

Effectiveness

May produce nausea.

Excellent for taking the
edge off the pain – it
still hurts, but you do
not care so much.

Crosses the placenta and can make your baby sleepy even
after birth, which can be serious if given close to delivery.
Baby needs to be closely monitored. May produce nausea,
which can be counteracted by another drug. You may be
confined to bed because of sleepiness, which, in turn, can
slow down labour.

Effective for women who are very
tense. Takes the edge off the pain.
Some find it a problem because they
can feel contractions but are too
sleepy to do anything about them,
such as changing position.

Administered by an anaesthetist. You must keep still while
it is administered, which may be hard during contractions.
You may need to be catheterized. A drip must be set up in
case blood pressure falls. Can slow contractions, so a drip
may be necessary to speed things up. Movement is
severely or totally restricted. You cannot feel contractions,
so may need to be told when to push. Risk of severe
headache if the needle accidentally pierces the sheath
around the spinal cord. Increases the chances of an
instrumental delivery (forceps and ventouse, see page 90).

The most effective form of pain
relief, which works in 90 per cent of
cases. Unfortunately some women
only feel the effects of an epidural
down one side of the body.

An anaesthetist needs to be available and you must keep
still. You are usually catheterized. Same risk of severe
headache as epidural. Movement is restricted. Nausea is a
common side-effect. Can take about five hours to wear off.

Very effective, fast pain relief for
unplanned caesareans and some
instrumental deliveries.

Medical pain relief
Gas and air or epidural?

If this is your first baby, you may have a number of questions about medical pain relief, in particular about gas and air and epidurals. Gas and air is suitable for both home and hospital births, and is considered safe for you and your baby, while an epidural offers the most complete form of pain relief. Questions may include whether the two forms of pain relief can be combined, when exactly during labour they can be used and what their precise effects will be.

Gas and air or epidural? **Common questions**

Q What is it like to use gas and air?
A Gas and air does not take the pain of the contractions away, but it will make you feel more removed from them. It takes about 30 seconds of breathing the gas for it to take effect, so it is important to start using it as soon as you feel a contraction building. It might make you feel woozy and light-headed, taking the edge off the pain but leaving you conscious enough to be in control. It can give you a dry mouth, so make sure you sip plenty of fluids. Bear in mind that using gas and air will restrict your movements to some extent, because you have to stay near to the supply, so it is wise to put off using it for as long as possible if you want an active birth.

Q Can I still have an epidural if I use gas and air?
A If you want to try some other pain relief, that is fine. Many women use gas and air while waiting for an epidural to take effect. If the epidural wears off close to the birth of your baby, you can use gas and air, which will help you feel more aware of your contractions.

Q When is the best time for me to have an epidural?
A You should really be in established labour before having an epidural, and if you have remained mobile for some of your labour you will have helped the baby to descend lower into the pelvis. There is no 'cut off' point for an epidural, as such: for some women it is still appropriate to have one, even if their cervix is 8 cm (about 3¼ in) dilated, because progress may have been slow and the baby may be in an awkward position. If you are in stage 2 of labour, and it looks as if you are likely to have a forceps delivery, a spinal anaesthetic may be suggested. This is similar to an epidural, but is given in a single dose. It takes around five hours to wear off, whereas an epidural wears off within an hour or two.

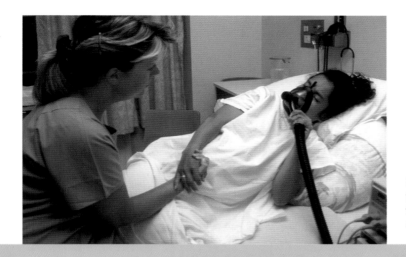

Left: Using gas and air, you will continue to feel the contractions, but at a slight remove.

Q If I have an epidural, how will I know when to push?
A It is better for your baby if you allow your body to do the work rather than actively pushing. Even with an epidural, the contractions will still move your baby down the birth canal – but it can take a little longer.

Q I am thinking of having an epidural for pain relief during labour. Does it hurt to have one put in?
A You might feel a sharp scratch as the local anaesthetic is injected into your skin before the procedure begins, but you should feel nothing more than that. Once the anaesthetic has taken effect, a fine plastic tube is inserted via a needle into the epidural space, next to the spinal canal. It can be 'topped up' from the tube, so there is no need for another needle. If you need an epidural in labour, then you are probably in pain anyway and the difficult part is keeping still so that the anaesthetist can carry

out the procedure. Occasionally the injection does not take effect, in which case the anaesthetist might try to resite the epidural.

Q Are there circumstances under which I would be refused an epidural?
A An epidural is not recommended if you have a blood disorder that increases your chances of bleeding, or an infection. Some spinal conditions, such as scoliosis (curvature of the spine) make it difficult or impossible to position an epidural.

Q Does a water birth mean that I cannot have other pain relief?
A Since it increases relaxation and reduces blood pressure, water may be all you need to help you with the pain. However, if you need something extra, you can use gas and air while you are in the birthing pool. Anything stronger than this would not be safe, so you will need to get out of the water.

YOUR BABY'S POSITION

Getting ready to leave the womb

The position of your baby in the uterus can affect labour and birth. By 37 weeks of pregnancy most babies will be head down, ready for labour.

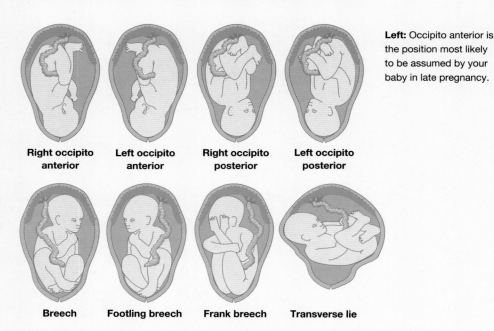

Left: Occipito anterior is the position most likely to be assumed by your baby in late pregnancy.

Right occipito anterior

Left occipito anterior

Right occipito posterior

Left occipito posterior

Breech

Footling breech

Frank breech

Transverse lie

The position of your baby is irrelevant until 37 weeks of pregnancy, as she will still be moving around. Even after 37 weeks a few babies are still moving, waiting for extra softening hormones produced at the beginning of labour before they engage. Others simply stay bottom down. A baby that is head down and fully engaged rarely changes position.

Occipito anterior

Your baby will probably be facing your back, with her back to one side of your abdomen. This

position is occipito anterior, or OA (the occipito is the back of the baby's head). According to the side of the abdomen on which the baby is lying, it is described as right or left occipito anterior (ROA or LOA). Most babies adopt this position, ideal for passing neatly through the pelvis: the baby can tuck her chin on her chest and turn slightly to emerge at birth.

Occipito posterior

The occipito posterior (OP) position is when your baby is lying with her back against your back, facing your abdomen. This may be right or left occipito posterior (ROP or LOP). Only about 5 per cent of these babies fail to move into an OA position. If your baby is one of the 5 per cent, it does not mean that you cannot have a vaginal birth. However, she won't be able to tuck her chin in so well and will have to rotate further in order to pass under your pubic arch. This is likely to make labour longer and to give you backache during labour (see below). Keep mobile, which will encourage your baby to turn, rather than having your waters broken.

Breech

A breech position is when your baby's buttocks are facing down and her head is under your ribs. Her legs may be tucked up (frank breech) or she may have one or both legs pointing down (footling breech). If your baby is breech, you may be offered an external cephalic version (ECV) at about 37 weeks. This is where the obstetrician manipulates your abdomen to try to turn the baby around (see Babies that do not turn, below).

Transverse lie

A transverse lie is when your baby is lying across your abdomen, with her head towards your left or right side. Unless she turns, you will need a caesarean.

Unstable lie

A baby that keeps changing position after 37 weeks is referred to as an unstable lie. Labour may be induced while she has her head down.

Babies that do not turn

If your baby does not turn head down spontaneously by 34 weeks, you could encourage her to do so (see box). Your doctor

Five steps to the **best position**

There are ways of encouraging your baby to get into the best position for labour.

1 Sit with your knees lower than your hips.
2 When standing, lean over slightly as much as possible, for example, over a work surface, thus allowing your baby more space to turn.
3 Swim – breaststroke is best – because the buoyancy gives your baby more room to move around.
4 Try kneeling on all fours as often as possible so that gravity helps the baby's spine, which is heaviest, to move round.
5 Adopt a knee to chest position for five to ten minutes four times a day.

might also try to turn her. This option should be discussed with you first. You will be asked to lie on your back with your knees up and relax while the doctor massages your abdomen. This is called external cephalic version (ECV). No force is used and the doctor will stop if your baby clearly does not want to move. After 36 weeks it is sensible to discuss breech birth with your midwife (see page 92) in case your baby does not turn. Only 3 per cent of babies remain in a breech position at birth.

Backache labour

If your baby is in a back-to-back (occipito posterior) position, you are more likely to have backache during labour. This is because the baby's head is pressed against your sacrum and the base of your spine. You can relieve the pain to some extent by getting into an all-fours position during labour, which makes the baby drop down, away from the spine.

Relaxing and breathing

Labour is a physical task, like running a marathon. If you run stiffly the race is harder. When your uterus contracts strongly, other muscles tend to join in, but if you relax it works more effectively and your body's natural painkillers flow. During labour you should keep checking so that you can release tension before it engulfs you: pull your shoulders down and let them go, part your lips to loosen your jaw, turn your palms upwards.

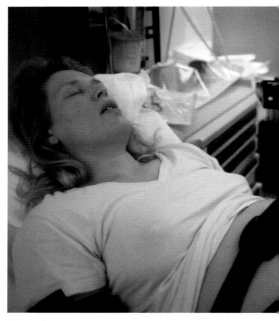

Above: Slow, deep breathing will help to keep you relaxed during labour.

Breathing techniques

Controlling your breathing will help you to relax.
- **Sit or stand comfortably, with loose shoulders, hands and face.**
- **Breathe in deeply through the nose and out through the mouth.**
- **Relax your body as you breathe out.**
- **Find something on which to focus as you breathe – your partner's eyes or an image in your mind.**

Relaxation and breathing are intertwined: if you relax deeply, your breathing will adjust to the optimum level. You already unconsciously change your breathing pattern according to what you are doing, for example, when drifting off to sleep, exercising or sinking into an armchair at the end of the day. Nobody had to teach you to do this; it is automatic. Likewise, any kind of stress automatically affects your breathing. It will become faster and shallower, from the upper part of the lungs, and will cause tension in your shoulders.

During labour, the majority of women find that the stress of being in an unfamiliar environment and coping with contractions makes them tense. Therefore you need to find a breathing technique that will keep you relaxed and tension free. When you feel Braxton Hicks tightenings (see box), practise taking slow, deep breaths, just as you will do when you are in labour.

Relaxing and breathing **Common questions**

Q What are Braxton Hicks tightenings?
A These mild, irregular tightenings are present from the beginning of pregnancy but you do not usually become aware of them until about the beginning of late pregnancy. These tightenings are named after the doctor who discovered their purpose, and they are a normal part of pregnancy. They squeeze blood out of the uterine veins, enabling them to fill with fresh blood, and help to stretch the lower part of the uterus, preparing it for labour. They do not mean that you are going into labour, but they do give you a good opportunity to practise your breathing techniques.

Q Can I use breathing to help me if I get the urge to push before I am fully dilated?
A Yes, panting through a contraction, or using gas and air, will help you to stop pushing and will reduce the pressure on the cervix. The best position to adopt is on all fours, with your head and chest down and your bottom in the air. Alternatively lie on your left side. Practise taking two short in-and-out breaths followed by a longer one: pant, pant, blow. Do not worry about forgetting what to do; your midwife will be there to remind you.

Q How should I apply the breathing techniques during contractions?
A At the start of a contraction, breathe in slowly and deeply through your nose. Hold for a couple of seconds and then breathe out slowly through your mouth. Try to keep your breaths the same length throughout the contraction. Your breathing will become a little faster towards the end of your labour, when your contractions become intense. This is fine as long as you do not start to panic and take very short breaths. Always concentrate on a long 'out' breath, as it is difficult to be tense when breathing out.

Q How can my birth partner help me with my breathing techniques?
A It is sensible to practise your breathing techniques with your birth partner before you go into labour. He or she will then be able to guide you during labour if necessary – you may temporarily forget to concentrate on your breathing once the contractions begin to get more painful! Your birth partner should also remind you to keep your face relaxed during labour. If your face is relaxed it is difficult to tense other parts of your body.

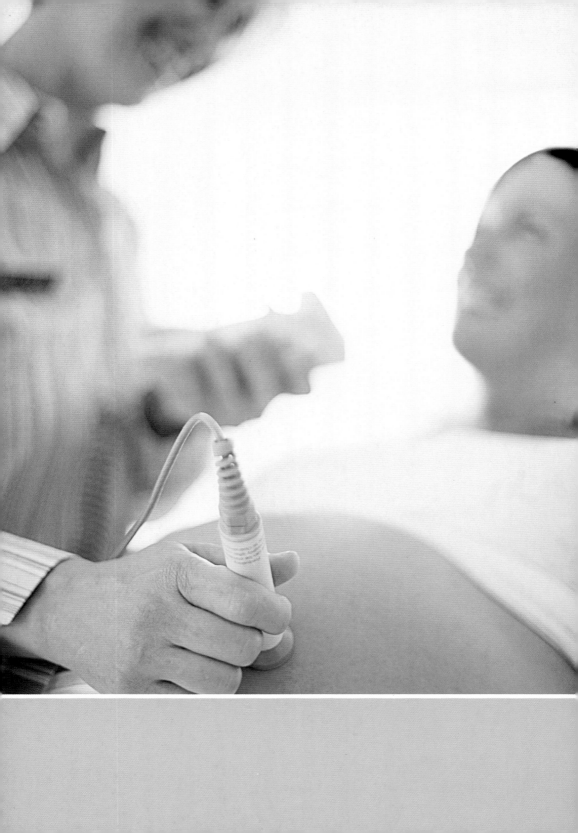

3

labour

Labour: an overview

The uterus consists of muscle, which tenses and relaxes during a contraction. At the bottom is the cervix, which also forms the top of the vagina. As part of the birth process, changes must occur in the cervix in order for the baby to pass through it and into the birth canal. The cervix will gradually get softer and thinner, and then it will start to dilate (open) in preparation for the birth.

The onset of labour

Many women have regular contractions as the cervix thins and the baby's head moves deeper into the pelvis. You may feel niggly pains that come and go over several days (latent phase of labour), or you may have painful tightenings that continue for hours, or even a day. The length and strength of the contractions is usually more significant than the length of time between them. If they last 30–40 seconds and you feel normal enough to chat or drink a cup of tea in between them, you are unlikely to be in established labour, even if the contractions are five minutes apart.

Established labour

The accepted definition of established labour is the onset of regular contractions together with dilation of the cervix. If you are getting contractions but your cervix has not started to dilate, this is still regarded as early labour (latent phase), which is different from established labour, which is the point of no return.

Established labour is divided into three stages:

- **Stage 1** – from the start of regular contractions and the opening of the cervix until the cervix has fully dilated (10 cm/4 in). With a first baby this takes an average of 10–12 hours. (See also page 64.)
- **Stage 2** – from full dilation of the cervix to the birth of the baby. When the cervix is fully open you will be able to push the baby down the birth canal. With a first baby, this takes an hour on average but it can be a lot longer. The second stage is often shorter in subsequent pregnancies. (See also page 76.)
- **Stage 3** – from the birth of your baby to the delivery of the placenta and membranes (the bag that contained the fluid surrounding your baby). This can last between ten minutes and an hour. (See also page 78.)

Labour **Common questions**

Q This probably sounds silly, but how will I know when I'm in labour?

A Many women worry that they won't recognize labour – but you will. Most labours start with mild, period-like cramps that gradually develop a pattern. Some mums-to-be feel it low in their stomach, others in the back. The latent (very early) phase of labour can last a few days, with aches and pains that start and stop. The general rule is: if you're not sure that you're in labour, then you're probably not! You might be experiencing the start of it, but when you have regular contractions that take your breath away, you'll know.

Q How long will early labour take and how can I prepare for it?

A This varies tremendously from one woman to the next. For some early labour may be just a matter of hours, while others experience mild, irregular contractions for days before labour starts in earnest. Try to enjoy the excitement of knowing that things are probably starting to happen, and pace yourself. Take a gentle walk, eat and drink as normal, and rest in the comfort of your own home. This 'pre-labour' phase can be tedious so make sure you have plenty to keep you occupied, such as watching videos, reading a novel, cleaning out a cupboard or addressing birth announcement cards.

Q Are there ways to make labour easier?

A Labour is easier if you have space to relax, and privacy so that you can let go of your inhibitions and flow with the rhythm of the contractions. Intrusions, or distractions such as moving from one place to another, may disturb this rhythm. Darkness or subdued lighting can help you to use instinct rather than rational thought. You need to feel safe and at ease in the place where you give birth, and with the people who care for you. Otherwise the delicate mechanisms of the natural birth process may be upset.

Q When should I start thinking about going to hospital?

A Staying relaxed is the key to coping with labour, and the longer you stay at home the better. A new environment is bound to make you tense and the labour ward is no exception. In general, it is too early to go to hospital unless your waters break (see page 73), your contractions are strong and five minutes apart, or if there is any bleeding. Of course, if you have any anxieties you can call the hospital for reassurance. You can also ask your community midwife to visit you at home if you are uncertain whether you have gone into labour.

Stage 1 of labour

The first stage of labour is the longest, lasting from the start of regular contractions and the opening of the cervix until the cervix is fully dilated (10 cm/4 in). It is then that the baby's head is able to pass through it. Although long, this stage is not relentless as, between contractions, you will have a break when you can rest, often for a couple of minutes at a time, even at the height of labour.

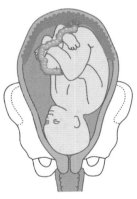

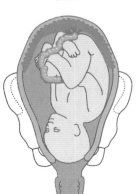

Left: During stage 1 of labour, the regular contractions move the cervix forward in your pelvis, soften it and make it thin out and open, so that your baby can pass through the birth canal during stage 2.

Because of the amount of stretching and softening that needs to take place, the longest part of labour is often the dilation of the cervix to 4–5 cm (1¾–2 in). Once you are getting strong, regular contractions, your midwife can perform a vaginal examination to establish just how far into labour you are. Most women lie in a semi-upright position on the bed while the midwife gently examines them using two gloved fingers. She can feel how far your cervix is dilated and also confirm the exact position of your baby.

There are a number of signs that suggest labour is not far off, but they do not necessarily mean that you will go into labour immediately:

• **A 'show'** This is a jelly-like, blood-streaked 'plug' of mucus that helps to protect your baby from infection during pregnancy. It often comes away from the cervix at the beginning of labour, although it can still occur a few weeks before labour begins.

• **Contractions** In the early stages of labour, these tightenings of the uterus feel similar to period pains, and you may also get backache (see page 70).

• **Diarrhoea** This may occur shortly before the onset of labour and can be regarded as nature 'clearing you out before the birth'.

• **Waters (amniotic fluid) breaking** This usually happens during labour with the force of a contraction, but it can also happen before labour begins. Most women find that their contractions start within 24 hours of their waters breaking.

Stage 1 of labour **Common questions**

Q I have been to classes and read all about labour, but I am not confident that I will cope when it comes to the real thing. What happens if I make a huge fuss?

A Women often worry that labour will be too big a job for them to handle, only to discover that they have hidden strengths. Relaxation and gentle breathing will help you to cope with contractions, so they are worth learning (see Breathing techniques, page 58). Also, remember that there are no rules when it comes to being in labour – all you have to do is let it happen. Relaxation really is the key to coping.

Q I hate internal examinations. Do I really need to have more?

A Nothing would ever be done without your consent, but internal examinations during labour give invaluable information about the progress of labour, and knowing what stage of labour you have reached can help you to make decisions about pain relief. Once you are in established labour you will be offered a vaginal examination, particularly if there is any concern over the progress of your labour. If you are nervous, share your fears with the midwife, or mention them in your birth plan (see page 22). If you don't want an internal examination, you don't have to have one, although you might feel differently once you are in labour.

Q I would feel so embarrassed if my waters broke in public. Is it likely, and if it happens what should I do?

A Fewer than 15 per cent of labours start with the waters breaking, and it mostly happens at home, where you spend most of your time. If you are upright and your baby's head is engaged, it acts as a 'plug' so usually there is not a huge gush but more of a trickle. Even if it does happen, it is unlikely that your baby will arrive immediately. If you are concerned, wear a sanitary pad when you are out. At home, put a plastic sheet over your mattress for the last month or so of your pregnancy.

Q What happens once my waters have broken?

A You should always tell your midwife as soon as your waters break. (If she is unavailable, ring the labour ward for advice.) She will check you over and listen to your baby's heartbeat. She may take a swab from your vagina to check for infection in case you do not go into labour soon afterwards.

Q Can I eat anything during labour?

A In a straightforward, low-risk labour, you should be encouraged to eat and drink as this will help to maintain your energy levels. Once you are in strong labour you will probably not want to eat very much. Some women find glucose tablets (available from most supermarkets) useful for maintaining energy.

Stage 1 of labour
Contractions

A contraction is when the muscles of the uterus tense and relax, passing in waves from the top, travelling inwards and downwards. During the first stage of labour, these muscles begin to 'take up' the neck of the uterus (the cervix), making it thinner and no longer tube-shaped. This process is effacement. Often the cervix begins to soften and move forward.

As these muscles stretch and relax, the cervix starts to open until it is fully dilated and the baby moves deeper into your pelvis. This completes the first stage of labour. During the second stage of labour, contractions play a different role, pushing your baby down the birth canal. After he is born, further contractions push out the placenta, which completes the third and final stage of labour. In the short term, the contractions vary in intensity, rather than getting progressively longer and stronger. However, overall, they become more frequent and last for longer as the birth approaches.

True story

Home birth with TENS machine and gas and air

'I decided that I wanted a home birth. A week before my due date I woke with mild stomach pains. I called my midwife Jenny and she said she'd pop in at midday. I didn't think I was actually in labour, but by 10am the pains were getting stronger. The gap between my contractions was rapidly getting shorter and I was finding it hard to breathe though them. Then, at 10.30am, I had a show.

'I still didn't believe I was in labour, but at midday I suddenly felt an overwhelming contraction. Luckily, Jenny arrived soon after and told me I was 4 cm (about 1¾ in) dilated. She called for a second midwife, who brought a canister of gas and air. I put on my TENS machine and started using the gas and air. Things progressed quickly. Just when I felt that the pain couldn't get any worse, my waters broke. The midwives said they could see the baby's head, and before long I felt it coming out.

'Suddenly Jenny told me to stop pushing and pant, as the cord was around the baby's neck. She managed to slip the cord over the baby's head and Breeanna was born at 3.10pm. I had a slight tear, but didn't need any stitches. It was fantastic to hold Breeanna and know I'd had the birth I wanted.'

Jaine, mother of Caelan and Breeanna

Contractions **Common questions**

Q How will I know when I am moving from early labour to established labour?
A To decide whether you are really in labour, compare your contractions with the ones you have been having. As they become longer and stronger, you will be more certain that true labour has started. Strong contractions last about 40–60 seconds, come regularly and definitely feel more purposeful.

Q When will the contractions start?
A Some women experience irregular contractions in the days before labour really kicks in properly, but none of this is 'wasted'. You may also experience Braxton Hicks contractions, which are 'practice' ones. They can feel irregular and uncomfortable, but they should not be painful. If you think that you are feeling contractions before 37 weeks, you should contact your maternity unit to get checked over, because at this stage your baby will be considered pre-term.

Q How much pain can I expect?
A Although a contraction affects the whole of the uterus, some women only feel it in one area of their abdomen or back. Most consider labour to be painful, but it tends to start gradually and build up, with the contractions intensifying as the cervix becomes more dilated. Some expectant mothers feel the pain through every nerve ending, while others find it easier to bear. After each contraction there is a period of rest, which helps you to relax and prepare for the next one. Contractions are temporary, and for many women it is this thought and the 'prize' at the end that helps them to cope.

Q What if my contractions slow down?
A Sometimes contractions can slow down or stop during labour, which can be quite disheartening. Staying upright and walking will encourage your contractions to keep coming. You could also try nipple stimulation, as this produces the hormone oxytocin, which can start your uterus contracting again. If that does not work, the midwife may suggest a synthetic form called Syntocinon, which is given intravenously (see Induced labour, page 72). If you become very tired or have an epidural, contractions are more likely to slow down. With natural childbirth, it can also indicate transition (see page 76), but there is a period of rest before the second stage of labour begins.

Stage 1 of labour
Positions

Although women in western countries have traditionally given birth lying on their backs, this is not the most effective position for either labour or birth. Women who remain mobile, adopt a more upright position during labour, or stand, sit or squat to give birth, generally have an easier time. Labour tends to be shorter, less painful and requires less intervention.

Best positions for stage 1 of labour

During stage 1 of labour, your cervix will be dilating and your uterus will be rising and tipping forwards. It makes sense to adopt the positions that will help these processes and assist in stretching the ligaments that join the bones of your pelvis.

Remaining upright, whether that means walking around or resting across a chair, will ensure that your baby's head is pressing on your cervix. This will encourage contractions, speed up dilation of the cervix and move your baby's head down and deeper into the pelvis. Imagine carrying a dining table through a doorway. It would need to be tilted from side to side, in the same way that your baby needs encouragement to descend through the pelvis. Changing positions and walking around can help her to move further down.

When you are having contractions during this stage of labour, it is a good idea to adopt

Positions for labour

In the last weeks of your pregnancy, practise these positions a couple of times to see how they feel. You will find out which are the most comfortable when you are in labour. You should move between them as your body dictates, with your birth partner's help if you need it.

- Sit halfway back on a chair, with your knees apart and leaning onto your birth partner for support and reassurance.
- Kneel on something soft, such as a large flat cushion or a folded blanket, spreading your knees to make space for your bump and leaning onto your hands. This position is good for stretching your pelvic ligaments. Rocking yourself gently in this position can help to turn your baby if she is facing forwards.
- Kneel on something soft and lean into your birth partner's lap with your thighs either side of his or her feet. You could also adopt this position leaning onto an armchair or your bed.

positions where you are leaning forwards so that your contractions work with gravity rather than against it, pushing your uterus forwards. Positions in which your thighs are braced and wide apart help to open your pelvis, so that there is more room for your baby to manoeuvre. Standing and leaning over a worktop, or into your partner, is an excellent position for encouraging labour.

Positions **Common questions**

Q Why is it so important to stay mobile?
A In stage 1 of labour, it is important to walk about as much as you can between your contractions. Keeping mobile will affect the speed of the contractions, your ability to cope with them and also the progress of the labour. On the whole, women who keep mobile during stage 1 have shorter labours and require less pain relief.

Q What happens if my contractions start during the night?
A If you go into early labour during the night, there is no need to leap out of bed and start pacing around. This will only tire you out. It is more important to go into labour rested and with sufficient energy to see you through the next few hours.

Q What is the best position to adopt if I want to take a break from moving around?
A When you feel like resting rather than moving around, it is better to opt for a chair than a bed or an armchair. Pad the seat with a pillow and sit back to front, with your legs either side of the chair back. Relax onto another pillow placed under your chin. Alternatively, kneel down and lean into a beanbag, or pillows if using the bed.

Q What should I do if I have a contraction while mobile?
A When a contraction comes while you are walking around, stand with your hands around your birth partner's neck, lean forwards and let him or her support some of your weight in a reassuring hug until the pain subsides. You can also support yourself by leaning against a wall, worktop or piece of heavy furniture.

'Keeping mobile during labour was fantastic. I could pace my own labour. When I stood up the contractions were strong and regular and when I sat down they slowed down. I felt totally in control.'
Nessy, mother of Gemma

Right: Your birth partner can support you as you find the most comfortable positions.

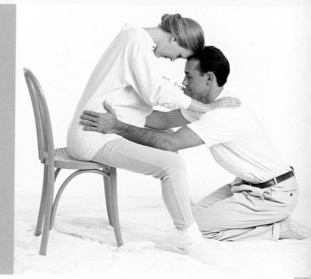

Unusual labour

There are times when the birth does not go quite according to plan. Some babies appear before time and rapidly, while others take a lot longer than average. Whether it is your first or your fifth baby, you do not know beforehand what your labour will be like.

What can happen?

Prepare yourself for any eventuality and remember that the midwives are at hand.

• **Sudden and fast birth** Labour can progress so quickly that the baby is born unexpectedly at home or on the way to the hospital. This is called precipitate labour and is unusual with a first baby. There are rarely any complications.

• **Long labour** About 80 per cent of first labours are over within 12 hours without any intervention. A long labour, although it can be normal, is hard to handle. It can be exhausting and demoralizing when there is little progress.

• **Backache labour** If your baby has his back positioned towards your back, it is harder for him to pass under your pubic arch during the birth. About 10 per cent of babies start labour in this position. Usually, the contractions gradually turn them into a better position for the birth. (See also page 56.)

True story

Taken by surprise

'As my first two babies were born safely and easily at home, there was no doubt where I wanted my third. There was little to worry about – same home-birth midwifery team, same birthing pool, same experienced father – so I put it to the back of my mind and focused on a work deadline in the week of my due date.

'My two previous labours had both been around four hours, so I knew we didn't need to call the midwife until I'd been having contractions for at least two hours. But the labour accelerated very quickly and my husband ended up catching the baby himself! Before he'd had time to wipe his hands he was on the phone to the ambulance men, who told him to leave the cord and keep the baby warm until the midwife arrived. She did shortly after – to a by then calm set of parents. The water in the birthing pool was very calm too, as I hadn't had a chance to get in.

'While I'd planned on a birth with the minimum of medical assistance, I hadn't quite had this in mind – but the elation and excitement afterwards were incomparable. They even gave me the energy to tackle that unmet deadline just a few days later!'
Tessa, mother of Lewis, Owen and Carys

Unusual labour **Common questions**

Q What can be the cause of a prolonged labour?

A There are a number of possible reasons for a prolonged labour, including the size of your baby and his position in the womb (see page 56). Contractions can also slow down if you are tense, if you lie down throughout labour rather than walk about, or if you are given pethidine or an epidural early on.

Q Is there anything I can do to speed up a prolonged labour?

A Labour can often be prolonged if you get tired, so it is very important to pace yourself and to keep eating and drinking during early labour, while you still feel like it. Being upright will help encourage the contractions to keep coming. Close contact with your partner – kissing and nipple stimulation – can also help to release oxytocin, the hormone that causes your contractions.

Q Will I make it to the hospital?

A Many women who have had a short labour the first time around worry that they may not get to hospital in time with their second child. If this is something that worries you, why not plan on a home birth? If you have a home birth the midwives will come to you, rather than you having to go to them. With a first baby, it would be unusual to have a very quick labour – but if that were to happen, just keep the baby warm until help arrives.

Q How should we handle a sudden birth?

A If you feel a sudden urge to push, get down on all fours with your bottom in the air and try to 'pant' through the contractions. This can delay the birth. If you cannot prevent the birth, make sure your partner knows what to do. Have a supply of clean towels to put under you and to wrap around the baby. If the baby's head is visible, your partner should encourage you to pant and 'breathe' your baby out rather than push. Putting his hand on the baby's head will help to 'control' the speed of the birth. When your baby's head is out, stay calm and do not try to pull out the rest of his body – it will come naturally with the next contraction. Your partner should carefully feel around the baby's neck and, if he can feel a cord, should gently loop it over the baby's head. Dry your baby with a towel to stimulate him if he initially appears to be floppy. Wrap him up, keeping the cord attached, and put him to the breast if you wish. If you feel the urge to push out the placenta after a contraction, do so, leaving the cord intact; otherwise leave it alone. Your partner should keep you and your baby warm until help arrives.

Induced labour

Despite their best intentions, some women need help getting into or speeding up labour, and it is best to be aware of this possibility, just in case it does happen to you. You may be advised to have an induced labour if you are overdue, if there is a chance of your baby becoming compromised or if the placenta appears to be no longer doing a good job of providing for your baby.

Induction for overdue babies

Women are normally offered an induction 7–14 days past their due date. Initially, an induction can take the form of a 'stretch and sweep', where the midwife gently inserts her gloved finger into your cervix and sweeps it around the bag of membranes. This can be done at your home or at the clinic. It can be uncomfortable, but it works in many cases.

If you are in hospital, the next step is to insert a pessary or a gel of the hormone prostaglandin into the vagina. This softens the cervix and can start the contractions. However, this process usually needs to be repeated, and it may be a couple of days before the contractions begin. Once the cervix has started to dilate, the midwife can break your waters using an instrument that looks rather like a crochet hook. This will be a little uncomfortable, but should not hurt.

If you still show no signs of going into labour, you may need an intravenous drip of Syntocinon. This is a synthetic hormone that makes the uterus contract. Such treatment requires close monitoring of both you and your baby because there is a danger of the uterus being overstimulated and your baby becoming distressed.

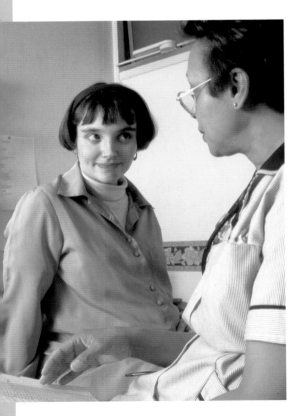

Left: If you are overdue or your baby is at risk, you may be advised to have an induction.

Induced labour **Common questions**

Q Will induction affect my baby?
A Most babies are unaffected by induction, but you will be monitored throughout to make sure of this. If the baby shows signs of distress, a tiny drop of blood may be taken from her scalp and analyzed to check her pH levels, which give an indication of her well-being. If necessary, she will then be born quickly. This test may be advised in any labour where 'fetal distress' is suspected, not just in inductions.

Q Does being induced hurt?
A How painful you find induction depends on how easy it is to establish your contractions. If you are overdue, or have given birth before, it may be no more than mildly uncomfortable. It can be painful if your uterus is not ready for labour. Pain relief is always available.

Q Should my waters be broken?
A It is now thought best to let the membranes (bag of waters) break by themselves. Once they break, the baby's head, which was cushioned by the amniotic fluid, drops further into the cervix, which can cause stronger contractions. You may find that you and your baby can cope better without direct pressure on your cervix. There are times when it may be advisable to break the waters, for example, if labour is induced or needs speeding up. If monitoring indicates the baby is becoming distressed, the midwife may suggest breaking the waters to see if the baby has opened her bowels – an indication of distress.

Q Under what circumstances would I need an induction before going overdue?
A There are various reasons for this, the most important being concerns about the welfare of the baby or mother. For example, labour may be induced if your blood pressure rises, or if you develop pre-eclampsia (see page 13), although the initial approach is to try and lower your blood pressure by rest or medication. The size of your baby is another factor: a small baby, who does not seem to be growing at the normal rate, may indicate a placental dysfunction, on the other hand, if you have diabetes, your baby may be getting too large. Finally, you may need to have your contractions 'kick-started' if you have not gone into labour naturally within a couple of days of your waters breaking, as this increases the risk of your baby developing an infection.

Q Under what circumstances would my labour be speeded up?
A Your labour may be speeded up if your waters break but contractions fail to start, if your contractions start but then stop, or if your contractions continue for many hours without progress. Sometimes the contractions are strong but fail to dilate the cervix, although they often become more effective if you can relax. If any of these apply, your baby will be monitored, and a hormone drip will be put into your hand to stimulate stronger contractions. The contractions may be more painful, but sometimes labour needs a kick-start.

MONITORING THE BABY

Checking on your baby during labour

A range of devices, suitable for different birth environments, enable the monitoring of your baby's welfare as labour progresses.

During labour the midwife listens to your baby's heartbeat through a handheld pinnard, a handheld Doppler or a cardiotocograph (CTG) monitor. The heart rate can change as the uterus contracts, returning to normal when the contraction ends and blood flows freely again. If a baby is becoming distressed, his heart rate can speed up or slow down too much, or return to normal too slowly, after a contraction. This provides an early warning of distress so that action can be taken straight away. However, towards the end of labour, it is normal for the heart rate to dip as he is being squeezed through the birth canal.

Monitoring different types of birth

How you and your baby are monitored depends very much on the type of birth that you have.

Active birth	• With an active birth, women are encouraged to keep upright and mobile as much as possible. This increases the likelihood of a normal birth (see page 68). As long as your pregnancy progresses without complications, you should be able to have as active a birth as you want without interference from continuous electronic monitoring.
Home birth	• Your midwife can use a handheld pinnard or Doppler but, if any complications develop and you need continuous monitoring, you may have to be transferred to hospital.
Water birth	• If you labour in a birthing pool, your baby's heartbeat can easily be monitored using a handheld Doppler. Some Dopplers are designed to work under the water but, if one of these is not available, all you need to do is raise your bump above the surface of the water so that the midwife can listen in. Even while you are in the water the midwife can lean over and do a vaginal examination, check your blood pressure, or whatever else is needed to monitor the well-being of you and your baby.

Different types of monitoring device

A variety of instruments are used to monitor babies, ranging from handheld devices to more complicated electronic equipment used for continuous monitoring.

Dopplars and pinnards

During your pregnancy, the midwife will have listened to your baby's heartbeat using a handheld instrument, such as a Doppler or a pinnard. A pinnard is a type of ear trumpet which she places on your abdomen and through which she can hear your baby's heartbeat. Many women prefer the Doppler because the sound is amplified so that they can hear the heartbeat as well. If your pregnancy has been straightforward and no problems are anticipated during the birth, research suggests that this is the best way of monitoring the baby's heartbeat during labour.

If your unborn baby opens his bowels (passes meconium), which can be a sign of distress, or if you are given certain medications, for example, an epidural or oxytocic drugs, it is considered safer to have continuous monitoring of the baby's heartbeat.

Cardiotocograph (CTG)

This instrument consists of two transducers which are held in place on your abdomen by elastic belts and connected to a monitor. The monitor provides a print-out of the baby's heartbeat and the uterine contractions. The monitor can be moved about so, unless you have an epidural, which restricts your movement, you can still stay upright or get out of bed. If everything is going smoothly, there is no need for it. However, there are many instances where continuous monitoring is

'I had to be monitored because of the epidural. But the CTG was like having a huge TV on in the middle of the room. We all just stared at it.'
Ceri, mother of Sofia

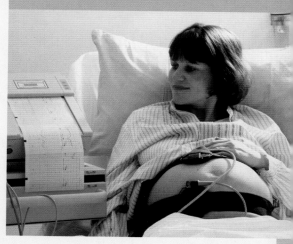

Above: A cardiotocograph (CTG) provides a print-out of the baby's heartbeat and the uterine contractions.

necessary, for example, during premature labour, if oxytocin or an epidural are being used or if the baby shows signs of distress.

Fetal scalp electrode (FSE)

Sometimes there are problems picking up an accurate and continuous reading of the heartbeat with the abdominal transducers, often because of the baby's position. In this case, it may be necessary to use an FSE. The midwife or obstetrician will carry out a vaginal examination to determine the position of your baby and then attach a small metal clip to your baby's scalp. This is linked by a lead to a CTG (see above).

Stage 2 of labour

The second stage of labour lasts from full dilation until the birth. The contractions, which are described as expulsive, are different from those in stage 1 and many women find it easier to cope with them. They cause an overwhelming urge to bear down and push out your baby, which is why women become more vocal at this stage, making involuntary noises with the effort of bearing down.

'I walked all through my pregnancy, and I walked miles during labour, too – round and round my bedroom, then the labour ward, then the delivery room. It was certainly an active birth, and really helped me with the contractions.'
Lorraine, mother of Poppy

The onset of stage 2 of labour can be confirmed by a vaginal examination, although many midwives find this unnecessary because there are often signs that the cervix is fully dilated. Other signs include:

• Involuntary grunting produced with the effort of a contraction.
• A heavy, blood-stained show (different from the show in early labour, see page 64).
• Bulging of the back passage.
• A slight dip of the baby's heartbeat with the contraction.

Transition

Many women experience a period of transition between stages 1 and 2 of labour. This can present itself in different ways. For some women it is a period of rest: the contractions ease while nature prepares you for the exertion of birthing your baby. Other women start to lose heart, begin to feel unable to cope and stop thinking positively.

Midwives often recognize this transition period and know that, with encouragement, it will pass. Some women vomit during this stage, which is another positive sign that they are approaching stage 2 of labour. Other women begin to get an urge to 'bear down', although the cervix may not yet be fully dilated. It is hard to fight the urge to push but you should be encouraged to 'breathe through it', and to turn onto your knees or lie on your left side, which will help to take the pressure off the cervix.

Stage 2 of labour **Common questions**

Q Will I open my bowels during this stage of labour?

A Many women have diarrhoea as a first sign of labour, and this is nature's way of clearing out the bowel before labour starts. A lot of women still open their bowels during the second stage of labour and, if this is going to happen, there is nothing you can do to stop it. 'Holding back' will only make you more uncomfortable. Even if your bowels do not open when you push, it will still feel as if they are, so you will probably not know for certain. During stage 2 of labour the baby's head puts pressure on the rectum, which is why you feel the need to open your bowels. This is a positive sign that the birth is imminent.

Q I have read that it is better to stay upright during stage 2 of labour. Is this actually true?

A Although many women give birth lying on their back, this is not an ideal position because you are working against gravity. It also places extra stress on the perineum, meaning that you are more likely to tear or need an episiotomy. Upright positions make pushing easier during this stage because your coccyx is swung back out of the way, giving your baby more room to move. (See also pages 29 and 68.)

Q What happens if I feel the urge to push too soon?

A If you push when there is still a rim of cervix in front of the baby's head, the cervix could swell like a bruised lip and take longer to dilate. Your midwife will guide you on what to do, but essentially you need to use gas and air or to breathe slowly through the contractions. Emptying your bladder can sometimes help to dissipate the rim of the cervix

Q How do I push?

A Women should not be coached in 'how to push'. It is better for you and your baby if you go with your body. You will bear down involuntarily and not hold your breath in the way that midwives have taught in the past. For the majority of women, the contractions in stage 2 of labour feel very different from those in stage 1, and this is because they are doing a different job. As your cervix is fully dilated these contractions have an expulsive effect, causing an involuntary, overwhelming sensation to bear down so that your baby is pushed out. Many women find this stage easier and do not need to be guided. They just go with their body and automatically push with the contraction.

Stage 3 of labour

The third stage of labour is the delivery of the placenta, which is expelled by the contractions of the uterus. There are two ways of managing this stage: naturally (physiologically) or actively (with an injection that speeds up the process). You should be given the opportunity to discuss the options beforehand, or put it in your birth plan (see page 22), but how it is managed will depend partly on the nature of the birth.

Natural management

Women who have given birth naturally, with no intervention, often want to complete the process naturally, without drugs. Once the baby is born, the cord is left attached until it has stopped pulsating, when it is clamped and cut. The uterus will contract naturally, but it can take longer to expel the placenta. Putting your baby to the breast and emptying your bladder can help to speed things up. Blood loss tends to be slightly heavier, but this is seldom a problem, as long as the mother is healthy and not anaemic.

Active management

Immediately after the birth, the midwife will inject a drug called Syntometrine, which contains oxytocin and ergometrine, into your thigh. This is a synthetic hormone that causes the uterus to contract and the placenta to detach from the wall of the uterus. You will feel a contraction and the midwife will place one hand on your lower abdomen while she gently pulls on the cord with the other hand. The blood loss tends to be lighter using this method, although the drug can make some women vomit. If you had an intervention during labour, for example, an induction, epidural or instrumental delivery, it is advisable for the third stage to be managed.

Stitches

After the delivery of the placenta, the midwife will check your vagina and perineum for any tears or grazes. A small tear that is not bleeding will heal naturally if kept clean and dry. A larger tear that involves muscle as well as skin may need stitching soon after the birth. You will

'During my pregnancy I used to worry about having stitches after the birth. When I tore, I was not even aware it was happening. The midwife put the stitches in as I was cuddling Annabel, and to be honest I did not give it a second thought.'

Sue, mother of Annabel

be given a local anaesthetic in the area before the stitches are put in. The stitches do not need to be removed as they will dissolve by themselves. If you have had an assisted birth (see page 90), the doctor will stitch the cut as soon as the placenta is out and while your legs are still raised.

The procedure for stitching is as follows. Your legs will be placed in stirrups with your feet higher than your hips. A local anaesthetic will be injected into the area a few minutes before stitching begins. The muscle is aligned and stitched first and then the skin. You may be able to use gas and air while you are being stitched, although the local anaesthetic should provide enough pain relief. If the stitching is painful, ask the midwife or doctor to stop until you are comfortable with the pain relief. The procedure usually takes about 20 minutes. At a home birth, the midwife will probably ask you to sit on the edge of a sofa or bed while she inserts the stitches, using a local anaesthetic.

Stage 3 of labour **Common questions**

Q With my first baby, I found that I remember shaking all over once the placenta was delivered. Why was this?
A It is perfectly normal to get the shakes after the delivery of the placenta. Your legs may feel wobbly as a result of a change in body temperature and loss of fluid, as well as the sheer effort of childbirth. All being well, you will now be given the chance to spend some special time with your baby, so that you can begin to get to know each other, before she is checked over.

Q I read somewhere that there were complications with active management if you have high blood pressure. Is this true?
A It is true that ergometrine can cause a rise in blood pressure, so, if you have high blood pressure, you will be given an alternative drug, which only contains oxytocin, intravenously.

Q What happens if the placenta fails to separate from the wall of the uterus?
A If various efforts to expel the placenta, for example, putting your baby to the breast and empty your bladder, have failed, it will have to be removed manually in an operating theatre. This procedure is undertaken under spinal anaesthetic and you would be given a course of antibiotics afterwards to reduce the risk of heavy bleeding and/or infection. It is important that the third stage of labour is not rushed.

Q When I gave birth naturally, the placenta didn't come out and had to be removed by a doctor. Why did this happen?
A A 'retained placenta' occurs in around 3 per cent of births. It can occasionally be caused by a midwife who, having given an oxytocic injection, pulls on the cord before the placenta has separated from the uterus. However, the placenta may also be retained even during a natural stage 3 of labour – it can often be just 'one of those things'.

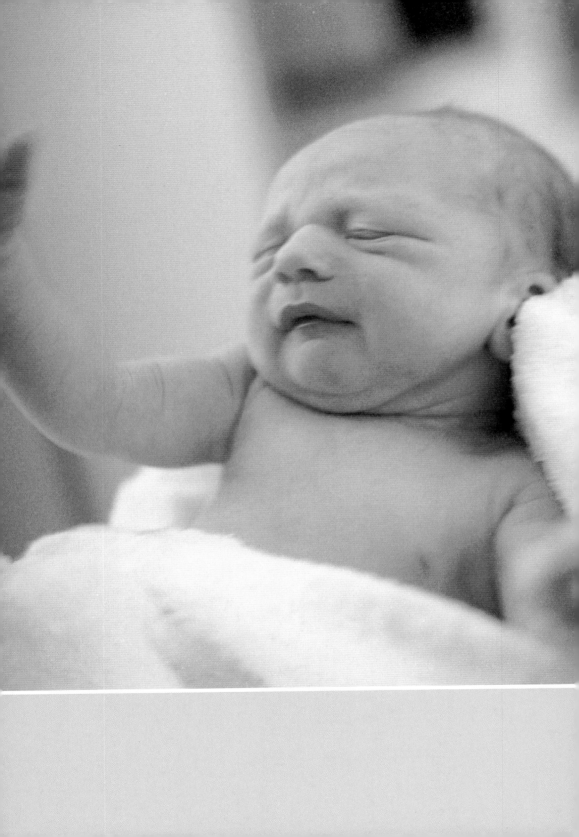

4

birth

Birth: an overview

Most women in stage 2 of labour feel an involuntary urge to bear down and push. You may find this urge scary at first, because it is so strong, but it is far less intimidating if you stop fighting it and go with it.

If you do this, you will naturally give three or four short pushes, of about five seconds each, with every contraction. Research suggests that going with your involuntary urge to push, rather than actively pushing, is better for you and your baby.

With each contraction, your baby will move down the birth canal until a small part of her head is visible. With a first baby, the head will slip back between contractions but it will eventually stay in position and more of it will be visible. This is called crowning. Some women experience a burning sensation at this point.

To control the delivery of your baby's head and to reduce the risk of tearing, the midwife may advise you to pant rather than push. Once the head is out, your baby will turn in line with her shoulders, which are turned to one side. The midwife will gently feel around her neck for the cord, which she can slip over her head.

The rest of your baby will be born with the next contraction. One shoulder will emerge from under your pubic bone. Your midwife will

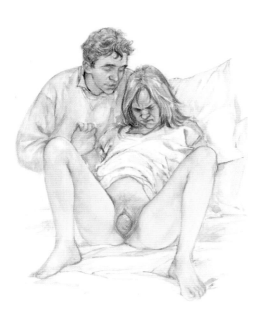

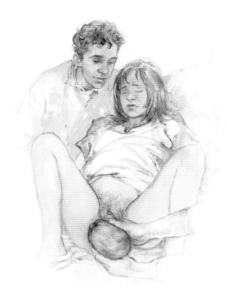

Above: Each contraction pushes the baby further down the birth canal, until crowning takes place.

Above: Once the head is out, the midwife will feel around the baby's neck for the cord.

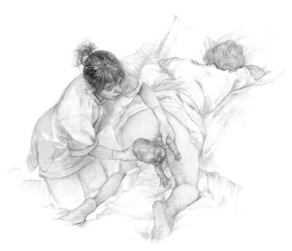

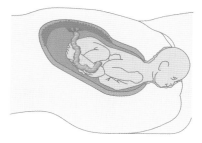

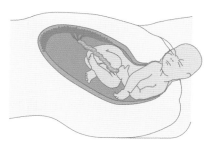

Above: Your baby's head will turn to come in line with her shoulders.

lift this and the head to give more room to the second shoulder. Then the rest of her body will slip out, with a further rush of amniotic fluid.

Above: The baby's head first crowns and then fully emerges.

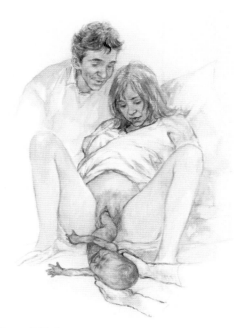

Above: With the next contraction, the rest of your baby will be born.

Five steps to help the birth

You can actively help the birth of your baby:
1 Choose the position that feels best to you at the time.
2 Visualize the progress of your baby, moving down the birth canal.
3 Remember that involuntary grunts are normal and can be helpful. Don't fight them.
4 Open out your birth canal and 'give' birth. Some women hold back for fear of emptying their bowels, a sensation that is caused by the pressure of the baby's head.
5 Try to keep upright and mobile for as long as possible.

Natural birth
Positions

There are a number of positions, including standing, squatting, kneeling and lying, that you can adopt to assist a natural birth. Your birth partner will be able to help by supporting you as you discover the positions that work best for you.

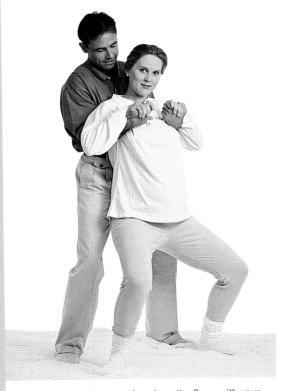

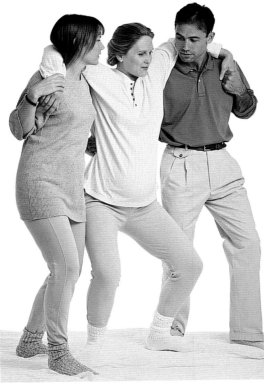

Bend your knees and push on the floor, with your partner standing behind you, with his hands under your arms for support. He can lean against a wall to support his back and bend his knees as you bend yours. Alternatively, he could support you from in front.

Stand or semi-squat, with support on either side from your helpers. As you push and bend your knees, your helpers should bend their knees too, taking your weight so that your feet remain on the floor, giving you something to push against.

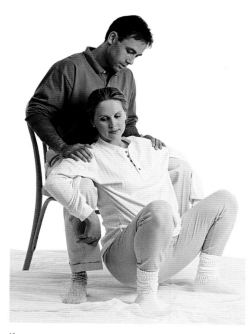

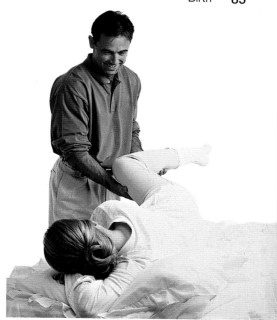

If you get too tired to stand, try this alternative. Squat between your birth partner's legs, leaning into his lap, with your feet placed flat on the floor and your arms over his knees. This position can be adapted for sitting on a bed, if you are securely propped up with pillows.

Lie on your left side with your knees bent, with your birth partner supporting your upper legs as you push into the contractions. This can be a good position for getting rid of the last (anterior) lip of the cervix.

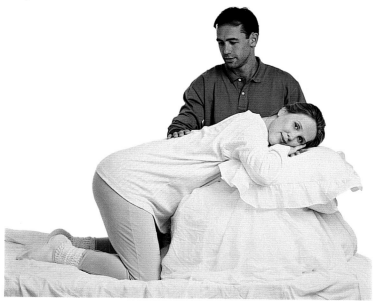

Kneel on the floor or the bed, leaning onto pillows or a beanbag. (You will feel more secure if you have something to push against.) The midwife can pass your baby to you from behind. You could also adopt an all-fours position, with your middle supported on pillows or a beanbag.

Natural birth

True story

Longing for a natural birth

'I wanted the birth of our second child to be totally different from that of our first child, who had been delivered by ventouse. Our community midwife, Jacqui, suggested a home birth.

'My due date came and went, but as my first baby was late I was not surprised. I booked an acupuncture session eight days after the due date and I do not know if it was a coincidence but 48 hours later I felt the first twinges of labour. At 6am, I woke up Tom and he arranged for his father to pick up our daughter.

'I put on my TENS machine and phoned the hospital to tell them I was due to have a home birth and to contact the community midwife. Fortunately, Jacqui was on duty that week and I knew she would be with us soon. So we waited, with the curtains closed and scented candles burning. Meanwhile, my contractions were getting stronger and closer together. I was relieved when Jacqui and her colleague, Wendy, arrived, and I put on some music to help me relax.

'Tom and I were coping fine, but it was reassuring that the midwives were there. At about 10am, I felt an overwhelming urge to 'bear down' and push. I tried all sorts of positions: on all fours, squatting, standing, but I found kneeling in front of Tom the best. I could hold on to him and being more upright definitely helped. All the time, Jacqui and Wendy were encouraging me. For the final pushes I sat upright on the floor against our sofa.

'Tom and I watched our baby's head appear – it was wonderful. We saw him turn and, with one more push, Jacqui was able to pass our baby to us at 2pm. She said we should have a cuddle and then tell everyone what sex the baby was. "It's a boy!" I shouted. Tom and I were overcome with emotion and even Jacqui and Wendy were crying.

'Tom cut the cord and wrapped our son in a towel. After a few minutes I was on our sofa, feeding Liam. I could not take my eyes off him. Now, when people ask me where he was born, my reply is, "Just there, where you are standing!"'

Rachel, mother of Liam

Natural birth **Common questions**

Q I want to have a natural birth but I am worried that the midwife might not let me. How can I make sure that I will be allowed to cope with labour in my own way?
A A large part of the midwife's role is to support you and be your advocate, helping you to achieve the sort of birth you want. Staying at home for as long as possible will increase the likelihood of a natural birth. Communication can be a problem when you are under stress, so write a birth plan (see page 22), discuss it with your midwife at your next antenatal visit and have it attached to your notes. If you are having a hospital birth, remind staff that you are keen to have a natural labour when you phone to say that you are arriving. Midwives can have different approaches, so ask for someone who will be enthusiastic about your plan – although all midwives should try to facilitate the birth experience you want.

Q How do hospital staff decide when to intervene and what help is needed?
A A midwife's training and experience tell her when help is needed. For example, she feels your abdomen to judge how your baby is lying. If she is unsure, she can confirm it once your cervix has started to dilate because your baby's fontanelle (see page 11) will be a different size. She takes your blood pressure and listens to your baby's heartbeat, judging whether they are normal, require close observation or warrant immediate intervention. Midwives are the experts in normal labour, so if either you or your baby is at risk, she will

consult a colleague or call in a doctor, who will decide what action is necessary. You will always be asked for your consent to treatment. She should also find out your wishes so that you can share in the decisions confidently and make an informed choice.

Q Can I touch my baby during the birth?
A If you want to, you can reach down and touch your baby's head once it appears. Many women find this helps them to focus on where they are pushing, as well as encouraging them.

Q Can I hold my baby straight after birth?
A You can ask to have your baby delivered directly onto your abdomen, if this is what you want. This is something you could put into your birth plan. You can take your baby naked, or cleaned up and wrapped in a blanket. The cord can then be clamped and cut, either by your midwife or your birth partner.

Q Will my partner be allowed to stay with me throughout the birth?
A If your baby is born at home, you can have anyone you wish with you. In hospital, your partner has no right to be present, but it is very rare for partners to be excluded. Most hospitals are happy to let you stay together throughout the birth, including during an assisted birth or a caesarean section performed under epidural. Many will not allow him to be there for a caesarean section under general anaesthetic. Most maternity units are happy for at least two birth partners to be present.

Episiotomy and tearing

An episiotomy is a small cut made at the vagina entrance to give the baby more room. In the 1970s it was routine procedure, particularly with a first baby. Today, it is given when the baby is showing signs of distress and a quick delivery is needed or when forceps are required (see Assisted birth, page 90).

What happens

Although it may sound daunting, once you are in labour episiotomy becomes much less of an issue. If you need an episiotomy, the midwife will first get your consent and then inject some local anaesthetic in the area where the cut is to be made. The area is very thin at the height of a contraction, and it is then that the incision is made – with one quick snip of a pair of sterile scissors. You are more likely to have an episiotomy if you need an instrumental delivery.

True story

A necessary episiotomy

'My contractions started on the Sunday morning. My midwife, Kate, popped round to check me over, and reassured me that my baby and I were fine and that she would return later. She was back at 2pm, and after a couple of hours I was getting an overwhelming urge to bear down. I just knew the baby was ready to be born. Kate kept listening to the baby's heartbeat with her handheld Doppler, and towards the end of labour it started to get slower. This is normal, apparently, as the baby gets squashed travelling down the birth canal.

'I remember a burning sensation as the head started to crown, and Kate telling me that I needed to push, as the baby was getting tired. I kept pushing and still no baby! Kate told me that she needed to do an episiotomy and I didn't question it – I trusted her implicitly. A few seconds later our beautiful Gracie was born.

'I never even felt the cut as it was done with a contraction, and Kate had applied some local anaesthetic to the area. She explained that she'd only ever had to do two episiotomies, but my baby was showing signs of distress and needed to be born as quickly as possible. I sat on the edge of the sofa cuddling my gorgeous new baby while Kate stitched the cut. It soon healed, with the help of a few lavender baths, and was a small price to pay for our beautiful daughter!'
Sarah, mother of Gracie

Episiotomy and tearing **Common questions**

Q Is it possible to prevent tearing?

A Nobody can guarantee that you will not tear because it depends to some extent on factors such as your baby's position and whether the birth needs assistance. However, there is some evidence that you can help to avoid damage to your perineum (the tissue between your vagina and anus) by gently massaging it (see below) from 34 weeks with sweet almond or wheatgerm oil. Practising your pelvic floor exercises (see page 112) will help you to become more aware of the area and relax it when it comes to pushing out your baby. As the baby's head is delivered, the midwife may ask you to 'breathe', not push, in order to control the speed at which the head is delivered and to reduce the chance of tearing.

Q My friend was really uncomfortable the first week after she had an episiotomy. Is it always like that?

A Usually yes, but there are exceptions and there's a lot a woman can do to help herself. Sitting on a special cushion that has a dip in the middle will help you to avoid putting pressure on the sore area, and lavender oil in the bath can make it feel more comfortable. Restarting your pelvic floor exercises as soon as possible after the birth will also help with healing, as it increases blood flow to the area.

Q Where am I most likely to tear?

A The most common tear goes from the entrance of your vagina towards your back passage. This area is called the perineum. A first-degree tear involves only the skin; a second-degree tear involves skin and muscle; while a third-degree tear, which is less common, involves the lining or muscles of the back passage. Sometimes tears are towards the labia or clitoris, and these can be extremely sore, particularly when you are passing urine.

Q If I need stitches after the birth, is it possible that they might burst open when I next open my bowels?

A Opening your bowels will not burst your stitches, but straining can make them feel uncomfortable – so make sure you try to open your bowels in the first two to three days after the birth. To avoid constipation, drink plenty of water, eat fresh fruits and vegetables and start your pelvic floor exercises.

Massaging your perineum

In the last few weeks of pregnancy, massage sweet almond oil or wheatgerm oil into your perineum for about five minutes each day. Immediately after your bath is a good time.

Assisted birth

Ventouse and forceps are both types of assisted, or instrumental, delivery, in which instruments are used to assist with the birth of the baby. An obstetrician will perform both types of delivery. They can only be used during stage 2 of labour, so if your baby needs to be born quickly before this stage, he would be delivered by emergency caesarean section (see page 94).

'I never wanted a forceps delivery but when the midwife told me that the baby's heartbeat was slowing down because he was becoming distressed, I just wanted him to be born. I didn't care how. My birth plan went out the window but I was so relieved that David was all right that nothing else seemed important.'
Yvonne, mother of David

Ventouse/forceps trial

The obstetrician will carry out a vaginal examination in order to decide on the most appropriate instrument to help deliver your baby. This will depend on the position of the baby and how far down the birth canal he is. If there is a significant chance of the instrumental delivery failing, you will be advised to have the procedure in the operating theatre, where the obstetrician can quickly and easily proceed to a caesarean section. This is called a trial of ventouse/forceps. Your bladder will be emptied prior to the procedure, using a catheter, and your legs will be placed so that your feet are higher than your hips. Your midwife will stay with you throughout.

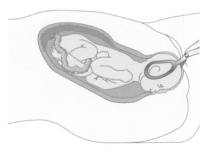

Above: Forceps cradle the head, guiding and lifting the baby out.

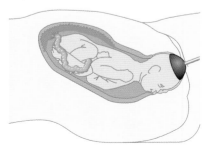

Above: A ventouse uses suction to help guide the baby through the birth canal.

Assisted birth **Common questions**

Q Under what circumstances would I need an assisted birth?

A This type of birth is commonly used if you have been pushing for a long time and your baby is making slow progress down the birth canal, particularly if he is showing signs of distress. This is more likely if progress has been slow during stage 1, perhaps indicating that you have a large baby or that the head is not in an occipito anterior (OA) position (see page 56).

Q How does a ventouse work?

A A ventouse uses suction to help guide your baby out, and a metal or plastic cup is placed on your baby's head. The cup gets its suction either from a separate machine via a tube or from a handheld device. While you push with each contraction, the obstetrician will gently pull the cup, guiding your baby out. It is not always necessary to have an episiotomy with this procedure.

Q What are forceps?

A Forceps are a pair of metal instruments that look rather like two large salad-servers. They link together and are placed inside the vagina. The forceps cradle the baby's head and guide him out, although you still need to push with the contractions. Forceps known as Kielland's are used to help turn your baby if he is facing the wrong way. Otherwise, Neville Barnes' or Wrigley's forceps are used to guide and lift your baby out. Episiotomy is nearly always necessary if forceps are used.

Q What are the effects of an assisted birth on my baby?

A The birth can cause distress or trauma to your baby, so it is usual to have a paediatrician in the room with a resuscitaire (see Hospital birth, page 26). In any case, you may be having an assisted birth because your baby was already showing signs of distress, so it is a wise precaution to have a paediatrician and equipment to hand. Babies who have had a ventouse delivery commonly have a bump on the back of their heads. This is usually reddish purple in colour and can be quite prominent. Forceps can sometimes leave two red marks on the side of your baby's head, but any bruises or bumps should go down within the first week. Because of the bruising, these babies are more likely to develop jaundice. Occasionally, a baby will appear to be irritable after an instrumental delivery, so it is best not to let too many different people handle him initially.

Q What will be the effects of an assisted birth on me?

A Some assisted births are easy: the baby is simply lifted out, and the mother feels much the same as she would after a natural birth. Others are very hard work for everyone concerned. This is sometimes unavoidable, and you may feel considerably bruised and sore afterwards. You will be grateful that your baby is safe but may also feel distressed at what happened, even though it solved a problem and was not your fault.

Breech babies

Breech babies sit upright in the uterus rather than adopting a head-down position. About one baby in four is breech at 28 weeks, but only one in 40 at birth. Most have turned round by 36 weeks (see Your baby's position, page 56).

A breech baby can pose a simple mechanical problem at the birth. Usually the baby's head, the largest part, passes through the pelvis and birth canal first. The baby gets oxygen through the cord until her head and chest are born and she can breathe. The rest of her body, being smaller, slips out easily.

If her bottom emerges first, the cord can be compressed (reducing her oxygen supply) while her head passes through your pelvis. There must always be plenty of room for her

'It was a shock in labour when the midwife did a vaginal examination and said she could feel the baby's bottom, not his head. All along, everyone had been convinced he would be head down.'
Paula, mother of John

head to follow the body easily, because she relies on oxygen from the cord until her head is born and she can breathe. If your pelvis is roomy and your baby is of average size and well positioned, there is unlikely to be any delay during the birth. Otherwise, a caesarean section may be preferable to risking a vaginal birth that might cause her distress.

The procedure

In hospital, you will probably be advised to have blood taken for cross-matching and a drip or tube inserted for fluids, saving precious time in an emergency. Your baby may be monitored continuously (see page 74). Some breech babies pass meconium (open their bowels). This is usually no cause for concern.

During a breech labour, you may have more examinations to check dilation because your baby's bottom might slip through your partly dilated cervix, making you want to push too soon. A 'managed' breech birth is usually performed by a registrar, with you lying on your back with your feet in stirrups. You may be given an episiotomy to create extra room. Some doctors use forceps to deliver the baby's head steadily; others cradle it in their hands to keep it well flexed. Then everything should proceed like any other birth.

Women wanting a breech birth without intervention often give birth on their hands and knees, allowing gravity to assist the birth. Labour should be allowed to start and progress naturally, without oxytocic drugs. Little progress during labour would be an indication for a caesarean section.

Breech babies **Common questions**

Q What should I do if I feel the urge to push too soon?

A Some doctors suggest an epidural to reduce this urge. Other options are: using gas and air, kneeling with your chin on your chest so that gravity takes the baby away from the cervix, or slowly and sharply blowing out – as if you were blowing out candles on a cake, one by one – to stop yourself pushing too soon.

Q How will the doctors know whether it is safe to attempt a normal birth?

A At one time, X-rays or CT (computerized tomography) scans were used to help judge the chances of a trouble-free birth. A pelvic diameter of 11 cm (about 4½ in) would be considered adequate if the baby was small, while a large baby would need more room. This seldom happens nowadays. A scan may be performed before or during early labour in order to determine your baby's exact position, and you may be induced around your due date so that your baby's head is still soft enough to pass easily through your pelvis. If you have had a previous vaginal birth, the midwife or doctor may feel more confident in your ability to give birth to a breech baby.

Q What should I do if I know that my baby is breech and my waters break?

A A baby's bottom does not fill the pelvis, so contact your midwife straight away if your waters break. Otherwise, there is a small risk of the cord becoming prolapsed.

Q My midwife thinks I could have a normal birth for my breech baby, while my consultant recommends a caesarean. Whose advice should I take?

A A caesarean section is preferable to a difficult breech birth, so it depends on your individual circumstances. Research suggests that it is not necessary to deliver all breech babies by caesarean, so ask your consultant why he thinks it is necessary in your case. If you are unhappy with his answer, you could ask to be referred for a second opinion from someone who delivers breech babies vaginally unless there is a particular reason not to do so. Some midwives have handled many breech births and may feel confident in your ability to give birth naturally – often advising an 'all fours' position.

Q Under what circumstances would I need to have a caesarean?

A You would probably be advised to have a caesarean section if your baby was in a breech (and not a 'frank breech') position, was considered to be quite large, and was your first baby. Collect as much information as you can in order to make a decision about your care. If your baby was not found to be in a breech position until you were already in labour, you might be advised to have an emergency caesarean, unless it was too late and the birth was imminent.

Birth by caesarean

A caesarean section is a major operation involving an incision through the skin and muscles of your abdomen, and into the uterus, in order to deliver your baby. Unless there are medical grounds that make it the safest form of delivery for your baby, electing to have a caesarean is not a decision to take lightly. In the majority of cases the recovery time is much longer after a caesarean section.

When you might need a caesarean section

Some pregnancy and birth complications mean that a caesarean is essential. In these cases, the operation will be elective (see above) and will allow your baby to spend the optimum time in the uterus. These complications include:

- **Placenta previa** – where the placenta is low-lying and obstructs the cervix.
- **Placental abruption** – where the placenta detaches from the uterine wall.
- **Pelvic disproportion** – where the baby's head will not fit through the mother's pelvis.
- **Difficult position of the baby,** such as a breech or transverse lie (lying across the uterus). (See page 56.)
- **Twins or multiples,** particularly if one is lying in a difficult position.
- **Health problems** with the mother or baby.

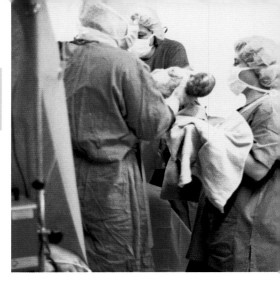

Above: The baby will be lifted out, shown to you and then checked over by the paediatrician or midwife.

There are three types of caesarean section, depending on when the decision to perform the operation is made (the surgical procedure is always the same).

1 Elective – where the decision to have a caesarean section is made before labour. There are many reasons for such a decision, for example: a breech position of the baby (see page 56), previous caesarean, active herpes in the mother, or the mother's pelvis being deemed too small for the baby's head.

2 Emergency – where the caesarean is unplanned. In this case, the baby may have started to show signs of distress in early labour, or there has been very little progress. One reason for a decision at this stage is the discovery, after labour has started, that the mother's pelvis is too small for the baby's head to pass through.

3 Crash – which is a true emergency. If the mother does not already have an epidural in place, she would need a general anaesthetic because the baby needs immediate delivery. Reasons for this include placental abruption, a prolapsed cord or severe signs of distress shown by the baby's heartbeat.

True
story

An elective caesarean

'I'm a great believer in natural, active births and I'd decided that my home birth was going to be as natural as possible, with no medical intervention unless completely unavoidable. I felt the first twinge of a contraction at 11pm, nine days after my due date. By morning the contractions were stronger but I felt focused, prepared and calm, remembering the advice I'd been given at an inspiring workshop about dealing with each contraction as it came. The homeopathy labour kit that I'd bought was being put to good use, as were the aromatherapy candles and music for maintaining a pleasant, relaxed atmosphere. The day passed. And the next. The baby's heartbeat was constantly monitored and was fine.

'The contractions increased in intensity over the days and were sometimes acutely painful, but I was able to deal with them naturally, without resorting to pain relief. My husband had taken the week off work and my mum was administering hot towels to my lower back, by far the most effective form of natural pain relief I used.

'I entered the third day of labour tired but hopeful. An internal examination by one of my midwives revealed that I'd only dilated to 4 cm (about 1¾ in). Feeling sure that the end of the first stage of labour must be approaching, I persevered. By the end of the day, however, I started to suspect that something was wrong. I spent a while going though the options with my husband and the midwives, and we decided that I should go to the hospital. I was too tired to be disappointed.

'At the hospital I was wired up and given Syntocinon, which didn't do much apart from making my contractions more regular. The baby was monitored and was fine. But I wasn't! After 75 hours of labour I knew I'd done my best, but enough was enough and I was content for the professionals to take over.

'The doctors and midwives suggested an emergency caesarean section as the baby's head was getting bruised because my contractions were so strong and she wasn't budging. I really didn't think there was another option, as I'd given it my best shot, and at 1.51am my little daughter was delivered to the delight and relief of us all.'

Ellie, mother of Anneke

Birth by caesarean
The operation

A caesarean section is no different from any other operation and you should remove all jewellery and nail polish. The top of your pubic hair will be shaved off, and the midwife will insert a catheter into your bladder just prior to the operation.

A needle will be put into your hand through which fluid will drip in case your blood pressure drops. It takes about ten minutes from the first incision until the birth of your baby, and about another 40 minutes for the stitches to be put in the layers of muscle, fat and skin. The procedure will not hurt, but you will be aware of the pushing and pulling inside of you. Some women describe it as 'someone washing dishes inside their stomach'. The scar is just below the bikini line and will fade in time. (See also Caesarean recovery, page 116.)

Birth by caesarean **Common questions**

Q What are the advantages of an elective caesarean section?

A With an elective caesarean, you know when your baby will be born, and you and your partner can both plan for the birth. You will avoid the pain of contractions, as the operation usually occurs before you go into labour, and there is less strain on the pelvic floor muscles. There will be no need for an episiotomy (see page 88).

Q What are the disadvantages?

A Medical evidence shows that, unless there are health issues that outweigh the risks, a caesarean is not as safe for mother and baby as a normal birth. It is a major surgical procedure with a recovery period of at least six weeks, during which time you should not drive or lift heavy weights. There can be complications, such as wound infection or poor healing, and there can be serious long-term consequences, such as reduced fertility. You will spend longer in hospital after a caesarean – usually around five days. You may avoid the pain of labour but you will have pain after the surgery.

Q What should I pack for an elective caesarean section?

A Big knickers are essential after a caesarean section, as you will have a wound along the top of your pubic line, just where the top of bikini-style knickers sits. You will also need sanitary towels, as you will bleed afterwards. You should also be prepared for a longer than usual stay in hospital (see above).

Q What kind of anaesthetic will be used?

A You will usually be given a spinal block or epidural so that you can stay awake during the operation and hold your baby soon afterwards. A general anaesthetic may be advisable if any

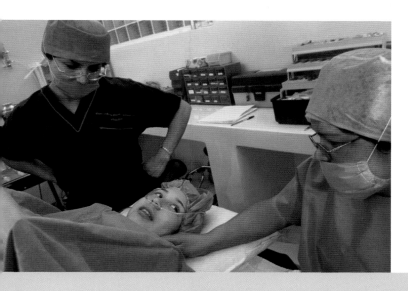

Left: A screen will be placed to prevent you seeing below your chest during the operation.

complications are anticipated, for example, if there is a risk of heavy bleeding, as with placenta previa. If you do have a general anaesthetic, it will be used for the minimum of time as it is better for your baby. You will therefore be awake in the operating theatre until the staff are ready to begin the operation.

Q What is the difference between an epidural and a spinal block?

A A spinal block, which is a single injection into the fluid around the spinal cord, is similar to an epidural, but tends to act more quickly. With an epidural, a fine plastic catheter is inserted into your back and left there so that the drug can be topped up during labour, either by an infusion pump or by the midwife. A spinal block provides a shorter but very effective dose of anaesthetic and usually lasts for about three hours. Because of this, spinal blocks tend to be used more often with caesarean sections.

Q Can my partner stay if I have an emergency caesarean section?

A In a true emergency, everyone would have to act very quickly and you would need a general anaesthetic if you did not already have an epidural in place. In this the case your partner would probably be advised to wait elsewhere until the baby was born and you were in the recovery room.

Q How much will my partner actually see?

A If your partner goes into the operating theatre with you, he will see very little. Once everything has been set up and the anaesthetist has put your spinal block in position, a screen will be placed across you so you see nothing from the top of your chest downwards. Your partner will sit next to you, so he can only see your head and shoulders (he could ask to look over the screen, but this may be discouraged). The baby will be shown to you as she is lifted out.

Twins and multiples

The majority of twins are born in hospital. Many are delivered vaginally without complications and you would be advised to have continuous monitoring. If a problem occurs, an assisted birth (see page 90) or a caesarean section (see page 94) might be necessary, even if the first baby was born normally.

True story

Twins!

'My husband Kevin was working away when the hospital confirmed the news that I was expecting twins. I felt petrified and cried buckets – Jack was only 14 months old and the thought of two more to care for was overwhelming. I had a difficult pregnancy. I was sick every day, and I developed symphysis pubic dysfunction (SPD) – a complication where the joints of the pelvis start to separate, causing acute pain. I also had antenatal depression. Fortunately my excellent consultant picked up on all my problems and made sure I got the support I needed.

'I had been given an epidural with Jack, which was an experience I did not want to repeat. However, my consultant would only advise a natural birth if I had an epidural in place in case of an emergency caesarean. As a compromise, I said I would start off with a TENS machine, but have an epidural once labour was fully established.

'In the event, the birth was a fantastic experience. I went into hospital to be induced and was found to be in early labour. A midwife broke my waters, Kevin helped me put on the TENS machine, and I was attached to a couple of monitors. After five hours I was fully dilated, although I had hardly felt a thing. Katelin was born almost immediately, then the midwife popped Charlotte's waters and she arrived just eight minutes later. Both girls were a good healthy size.

'Having twins is quite an experience. Perhaps the most surprising thing is that two children can be genetically identical and yet have completely different personalities: Katelin is very girly, whereas Charlotte is a complete tomboy!!'
Steph, mother of Jack, Katelin and Charlotte

Procedure

In some hospitals, it is policy for twins to be delivered in an operating theatre (even in the case of vaginal deliveries) or in a larger delivery room, for safety and to accommodate a midwife and paediatrician for each baby, as well as the obstetrician.

You may be advised to have an epidural because there is a greater chance of you needing a caesarean section. If your twins are delivered vaginally, the obstetrician or midwife will confirm the position of the second twin after the birth of the first and break the waters if necessary. The second twin may be lying across the uterus, in which case it may be possible to turn him into either a breech or a head-down position, so that he can also be delivered vaginally. Usually, you will be given a hormone drip to make sure that your contractions continue. The second twin is usually born within 20 minutes of the first.

Occasionally the second twin will show signs of distress, in which case you will be given an assisted birth or a caesarean section. You will usually be given a hormone drip after the birth. This encourages the uterus to contract and, given the large area covered by the placenta, reduces the risk of bleeding.

Twins and multiples
Common questions

Q How will I know whether I can attempt a vaginal birth or need to have a caesarean?
A Although there is a higher chance of a caesarean section than in a singleton pregnancy, many women still have vaginal births. It is possible to have a normal birth if the presenting twin is in a head-down position. However, if the first twin is in a breech position, your obstetrician will often recommend a caesarean section. During labour, an emergency caesarean may be required, either because labour is not progressing well or because there is evidence of fetal distress. Triplets or more are usually delivered by caesarean section. Much depends on the positions of your babies when you go into labour. Many women still choose to give birth naturally with the minimum of intervention, although you will probably be advised to have 'high-tech' management of the birth.

Q I am expecting twins. Will labour and birth be twice as painful for me as for mothers having just one baby?
A Giving birth to twins does not necessarily mean that labour will be any longer or any harder for the baby. In fact, because twins are born earlier and are usually smaller than average, the birth may be even quicker.

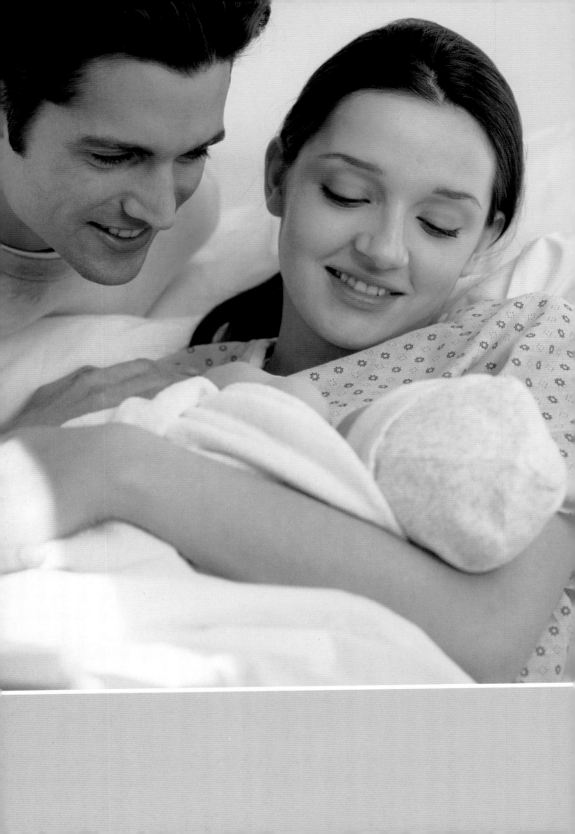

5

after the birth

You and your baby
Your first contact

Nothing can prepare you for how you will feel when you first see your baby. If you see her before the midwife has cleaned her up, she may be slightly blue and covered in vernix (see page 104), but she will still be a source of wonder. Remember to let the midwife know in advance if you want your baby to be placed onto your belly when she is born.

Contact

Try to have some skin-to-skin contact with your baby immediately after the birth, to start the bonding process. Cuddle and stroke her and give her an opportunity to smell and feel the warmth of your skin and listen to your voice.

If you have decided to breastfeed, you may want to put your baby to the breast soon after the birth. Babies have very strong sucking reflexes during the first hour and often latch on really well. Putting your baby to the breast also causes a reflex that helps the uterus contract, reducing bleeding. However, your baby may be too sleepy to be interested in feeding.

Some babies need an early feed to help boost their blood sugar level, especially if they needed any medical attention when they were born and used up a lot of energy to get their heart and lungs working well.

Below: Skin-to-skin contact with your newborn is just the start of the bonding process.

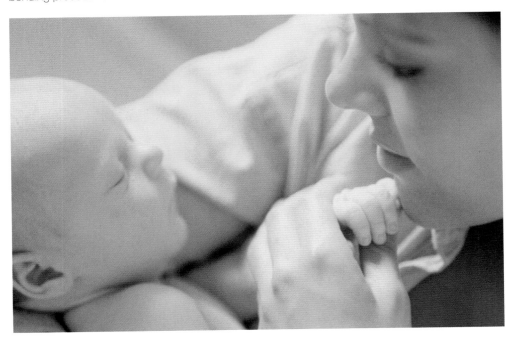

Your first contact **Common questions**

Q I am anxious that I will not know how to breastfeed my baby when she is born. Is there anything I can do?

A If you need help with breastfeeding the midwife will be there to support you. Once you feel confident, try putting your baby to the breast yourself and then ask the midwife to check that she is latched on properly. Some babies latch on immediately, but the majority need to learn what to do. At the beginning, you may find that your baby only takes a few sucks at a time. This is quite normal. She is discovering what to do, getting to know your smell and stimulating your breasts, which will help them to produce the milk (see also Feeding, page 122).

True story

First cuddles

'I finished work on a Friday and celebrated the start of my maternity leave by going out after work with my colleagues. Little did I know then that I'd be giving birth just hours later!

'With my husband, Bill, I'd decided that I'd like the baby to be given to me as soon as possible after delivery – I didn't want to wait for her to be washed. So, while I was lying propped up in bed, she was passed into my arms and soon got comfy nestling between my breasts. It was amazing to look down at this tiny baby, perfect and gorgeous in every way. I was overwhelmed. Not only had my baby arrived three weeks early, but I'd felt I was expecting a boy – and here was a girl!

'The cuddle that's really etched on my mind came four days later, though. Franchesca was slightly jaundiced and not breastfeeding properly. She was re-admitted to hospital on Tuesday and, after receiving phototherapy, she began to feed much better, but would cry inconsolably. I'd gone from feeling an amazing high to being really anxious.

'Then, at 4am, the midwife suggested I take Franchesca into bed with me. That's the moment I'll never forget. She calmed instantly, content simply to be cuddled up in bed with me. I watched her stretch, yawn and fall asleep with her arms above her head. Any worries I'd had melted away. I knew everything would be fine.'

Catherine, mother of Franchesca

Your baby's appearance

Beautiful though he seems to you, your baby may not look like the newborn babies featured in glossy magazines. Newborns are often blue, but their colour changes as soon as they take their first breath. They may be covered in vernix, the white lubricant that has kept them waterproof in the amniotic fluid, and they may be streaked with blood. If you had an assisted delivery, your baby may have marks or bumps on his head, which may be elongated or even lop-sided. All of this is normal and will resolve in time.

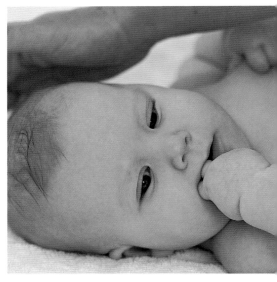

Above: A series of tests will be carried out during the first days of your baby's life.

The Apgar test

A baby's first check takes place at one minute of age. The Apgar test is repeated again at five minutes. Five categories are assessed, which are each given a score of 0, 1 or 2, the total being out of 10. A healthy baby will have a score of 7 or higher, whereas a baby with a score lower than 7 may need time to recover from the birth. A baby with a very low score may need medical attention. The five Agpar categories are as follows.

- **Appearance (colour)** Many newborn babies are not pink, but tinged with blue. However, they do pink up quickly after the birth. Non-

Caucasian babies are assessed by examining the inside of the mouth, the whites of the eyes, the soles of the feet and the palms of the hands.
- **Grimace (reflexes)** The baby should respond to stimulation, such as being handled.
- **Pulse** The heart rate should be over 100 beats per minute.
- **Activity (muscle tone)** The baby should be able to actively move his arms and legs.
- **Respiration** The baby's breathing should be strong and regular.

Early health checks

Within the first few days, the paediatrician or midwife will carry out a thorough series of checks. This is also something your doctor might do if he is visiting you after a home birth.

• **Head and neck** This involves checking the skull bones and fontanelle; the eyes, ears and nose; the roof of the mouth, to make sure that the palate has formed properly; and the neck for any sign of cysts.

• **Heart sounds and breathing** 'Innocent' heart murmurs may be heard in the first few hours as your baby's circulatory system adjusts. If the murmur continues, his heart may be scanned before you leave the hospital.

• **Spine** The doctor will run his thumb down your baby's vertebrae to check that the bones are in the right place and that there are no obvious abnormalities of the spinal cord.

• **Hips** The doctor will bend your baby's legs up and turn them out to check for signs of congenital dislocation of the hips (CDH).

• **Hands, feet, arms and legs** The doctor will check your baby's feet for signs of them turning in excessively (talipes). He will also look at the creases on your baby's palms – there are usually two. A single crease may indicate Down's syndrome. He will also check the muscle tone and strength of the limbs.

• **Genitals and anus** Babies commonly have swollen genitals after birth and a baby girl may have a vaginal discharge for a couple of days. The doctor will check that the genitals are formed properly and that a boy's testicles are in his scrotum and not undescended. The doctor will also ask you if your baby has opened his bowels (passed meconium).

• **Reflexes** The doctor will check your baby's reflexes, which are present at birth and indicate that the central nervous system is functioning.

Your baby's appearance
Common questions

Q What features should I be aware of in my newborn?

A It is quite normal for a baby's head to be swollen in places if there has been pressure on the head during delivery. He may also have puffy eyes. His head may look a strange shape because of the 'soft spot', or fontanelle, on top of his head, near the front. This is where the skull bones have not yet fused together (see also page 11). Any birthmarks will be pointed out to you, although it is quite normal for babies to have little pink marks, often called 'stork marks', which gradually fade. Some babies have a blue area on their tummy or back, a bit like a bruise. These are called 'Mongolian spots' and are often found in babies of African, Asian, Mediterranean, Native American and Canadian origin.

Q I noticed a mention of vitamin K in an article about birth plans. What is this for?

A Vitamin K helps blood clotting, and newborns do not have much of this vitamin. In rare cases, babies develop a problem known as haemorrhagic disease of the newborn (HDN), or vitamin K deficiency bleeding, which can be fatal. Therefore most babies are given vitamin K, either in the form of an injection after the birth or as drops into the mouth. However, this is your decision.

Hospital routines

Most hospitals have their own routines and procedures. Being away from home with your new baby can be quite daunting, so make sure you know what to expect and are prepared.

Midwife's checks

After the birth, the midwife will check you and your baby to make sure that you are both well enough to go home or, more commonly, to a post-natal ward. She will check that you are recovering well from the birth, that your blood loss is not too heavy and that any problems, such as a rise in blood pressure, are identified.

She will also want to see that your baby is thriving and feeding well, and that the cord is clean and dry.

Pamper yourself

Take some luxury toiletries with you to pamper yourself and a large fluffy towel for a bath or shower, as well as suitable clothes to change into (see What shall I pack? page 41). There is no need to sit around in a nightdress all day. When your partner visits, let him spend time with your baby while you soak in a bath and change into clean clothes. You are in hospital because you have had a baby, not because you are ill, so there is no reason for you to stay in bed.

Length of stay

How long you stay in hospital depends on a number of factors.

- **Type of delivery.** If you have had a caesarean section (see page 96) you will probably stay in for 4–6 days.
- **Blood loss.** If you have lost a lot of blood, you may feel a bit wobbly and may even need a blood transfusion.
- **Pre-eclampsia** (see page 13). If you have had high blood pressure during your pregnancy, it still needs to be monitored after the birth to make sure that it settles down.

- **Your baby's condition.** If your baby was premature and was taken to a special-care baby unit, you may want to stay in for a few days so that you can be close to her (see page 108).
- **Feeding.** Some babies take a few days to learn how to feed, either from the breast or the bottle.
- **Infections.** If you or your baby show any signs of infection, you may need a course of intravenous antibiotics, which will take a few days to take effect.

Hospital routines **Common questions**

Q How long will I have to stay in hospital?
A If you have had a normal delivery, you can usually have a wash or a bath on the labour ward, change your clothes, have something to eat and drink, then move to a post-natal ward. Some women choose to go home directly from the labour ward if there have been no complications – particularly if they have had midwife-led care and are confident about feeding their baby. However, women usually go to the post-natal ward after an hour or so and stay in overnight, especially if this is their first baby. The length of stay depends on the type of birth you have had and on the health of you and your baby.

Q Will there be someone who can help me with my baby?
A Nobody expects you to know what to do immediately. Many women have never even held a baby before and, not surprisingly, need help and support in caring for their baby. There are often nursery nurses or health-care assistants working on the post-natal ward, as well as the midwives, and all of them will be pleased to show you and your partner how to top-and-tail your baby, change her nappy, wind her and so on.

Q If I am tired, will the midwives look after my baby overnight?
A This does not tend to happen nowadays because it is much better if your baby stays with you at night. However, if you have been particularly poorly, a member of staff may offer to look after your baby for a while so that you can get some rest. Having your baby with you at night is part of the process of getting to know each other. Even if you feel very tired, which is inevitable, you will probably be more relaxed having your baby nearby, where you can see her, rather than wondering whether every cry you hear is hers.

Q Are there procedures for visitors?
A Once your baby is born, most hospitals prefer you to wait until you get to the post-natal ward before having any visitors. This ensures that there are not too many people wandering around and that the dignity of other women, who are still in labour, is respected. It also means that there will be fewer people in the way if an emergency arises. Once you are on the post-natal ward, your partner can usually visit at any time and stay as long as he wants. There will be restrictions on other visitors, for example, there may be specific visiting hours and children, other than your own, may not be allowed in.

Special-care babies

The special-care baby unit (SCBU) is a separate ward run by specialist nurses and paediatricians. These units deal mostly with premature babies, but there are other babies who also need to spend some time here. Especially after a full-term pregnancy, it can be a huge shock to parents to find that their baby has a problem that requires special care.

Parents can find an SCBU quite daunting, because it is full of beeping machines and alarms sounding on cots. Although the staff are used to this, parents tend to assume that every alarm is a sign of something seriously wrong, which is often not the case. Many babies have a fine cable attached to a pad on their foot or hand, monitoring their pulse rate and oxygen levels. If a baby moves or knocks against the pad, it may trigger an alarm simply because it needs to be repositioned.

Inside the SCBU

The majority of babies are born without any problems but, if there is any concern, they are best being cared for by specialist staff. There is a high ratio of carers to babies in SCBUs. The

Below: It is upsetting to see your baby in a SCBU; be reassured he is receiving the best care possible.

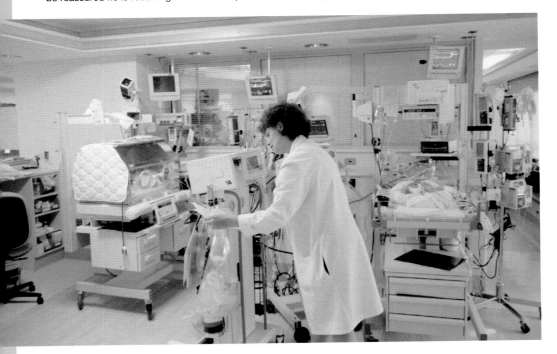

'I had never intended to breastfeed but when Jack had a chest infection and went to the special-care unit, the nurses encouraged me to breastfeed. I was so glad that I did this as I felt that it was something that I could do for him that nobody else could.'

Sally, mother of Jack

Coping with bad news

With so many screening tests available nowadays, parents assume that any significant problems or disabilities will be picked up during the pregnancy, but this is not always the case. Some medical conditions or disabilities, such as cerebral palsy, are not always identified before the birth.

Your initial reaction may be denial, thinking that the professionals have made a mistake. More commonly, the feeling is guilt. What did I do wrong? Did I eat or drink something to affect my baby? Although you will be reassured that you are not to blame, you will still feel guilty and blame yourself. It can help to get in touch with an organization where you can talk to people with similar experiences. These groups can be a great source of comfort, advice and hope.

Sometimes, despite all the efforts of the medical team, a newborn baby dies. Dealing with this tragedy is one of the hardest things parents ever have to do. It is important that both parents are open about their feelings of loss, so that they can learn to accept them and can support each other through the grieving process. If your baby dies, you will still be encouraged to spend some time with him, having cuddles and building some memories. You will be offered counselling, which can help to strengthen you in your bereavement.

care can range from a few hours of observation to intensive life support.

The specialist staff in the SCBU will encourage you to participate in the care of your baby and will explain what is going on so that you feel involved. Some babies develop breathing difficulties soon after birth, making a 'grunting' sound as they breathe. Initially a baby may just be observed and encouraged to have an early feed, but, if the difficulties persist, he may have developed an infection. In this case, the paediatrician will arrange for the baby to have screening tests, including a chest X-ray, swabs, lumbar puncture, and urine and blood analysis, and may also recommend a course of antibiotics. Some babies develop severe jaundice and need a course of phototherapy. Others have a very low blood sugar level or a structural abnormality, or they may have inhaled meconium during the birth.

How long a baby stays in the SCBU depends on the problem and how well he responds to treatment. SCBUs often have different 'areas' depending on the level of specialist care that the baby needs. As a baby improves, the staff will move him into other areas until he reaches the point when he is ready to go home.

Physical after-effects

If you look in the mirror after the birth and long for the instant return of either your pre-pregnant body or your bump, you are not alone. Remember that you have some way to go before you can feel in control of your body again. Not only have your muscles and skin been stretched, but you may also be retaining quite a lot of fluid (oedema). Your body needs time to recover after the birth.

Physical after-effects **Common questions**

Q My friend experienced severe after-pains following the birth of her daughter. What exactly are they?
A Once you have given birth, your uterus shrinks, eventually returning to its pre-pregnancy size. As it contracts in the first few days, you may feel 'after-pains', which are similar to period pains. These pains are stronger with a second or subsequent baby and are more noticeable when you are breastfeeding. Any pains should respond to mild painkillers, a soak in a warm bath or a hot-water bottle held against your abdomen.

Q My feet and legs feel swollen. Is there anything I can do?
A This condition is known as oedema and is the result of fluid retention in your legs. Raise your feet when resting or sleep with a pillow under your feet. You will gradually lose the excess fluid as you pass urine.

Q Is it normal to bleed after the birth?
A You should expect to have some blood loss, similar to a heavy period, even after a caesarean. This is known as 'lochia' and usually lasts for up to six weeks. However, the blood flow should become a lot less after the first week and will become more of a brownish discharge, gradually becoming lighter. Use sanitary pads rather than tampons, which can result in infection. If you notice any clots, show them to your midwife. She can examine them to make sure that it is only blood. Very occasionally, the clots contain a piece of placenta, which means that not all the placenta has been expelled. If the blood loss is very heavy, or smells bad, tell your midwife because this could indicate an infection and you may need antibiotics.

What can I expect?

When you consider the physical changes that your body has undergone during the processes of pregnancy, labour and birth, it is not surprising that some physical after-effects will be evident in the days after you have given birth. Don't worry: the following symptoms are normal and will eventually pass.

• Folds of loose skin and quite a 'bump' where your baby used to be. This will shrink and become firmer as the days pass.

• Tiny broken veins, bloodshot eyes, small bruises, piles or an aching pelvis, caused by the effort of pushing.

• Excess perspiration as your body gets rid of excess fluids.

• A slightly raised temperature for the first few hours around the third or fourth day when your milk comes in.

• Discomfort when sitting or walking; general soreness and exhaustion, especially after a difficult delivery.

Q I tore quite badly during the birth and find it extremely uncomfortable to pass urine. What can I do?

A Try passing urine in a warm bath, or pour a jug of warm water between your legs as you sit on the toilet. Drink plenty of fluids and resist the temptation to hold back the urine for as long as possible because this will make you more likely to get an infection.

Q How long will it be before my bowels are back to normal?

A It may be a few days before you open your bowels again. You may find being in hospital inhibiting and want to take your time in the toilet, and you may also be worried about any stitches you might have had (see Episiotomy and tearing, page 88). Make sure you drink plenty of water and eat lots of fresh fruit and vegetables, as well as other fibre-rich foods.

Also, remember that any codeine-based painkillers can cause constipation. If you still have not opened your bowels a few days after returning home, your midwife can arrange for you to have a mild laxative.

Q How long will it take to lose the weight I have put on?

A Women vary in the amount of weight they gain in pregnancy, and in the time it takes to return to their pre-pregnant shape. You will lose some weight almost straight away after the birth, and more weight is lost as the uterus contracts to its normal size. It is important not to do too much when you are a new mother, so rather than aiming to return to your pre-pregnancy weight as fast as possible, try to relax, feel good about yourself and be assured that, with all the exercise you get from looking after a new baby, you will soon lose weight.

Pelvic floor exercises

The pelvic floor consists of a 'hammock' of muscles and ligaments, resembling a figure of eight, and stretches from your pubic bone (at the front) to the bottom of your backbone. This holds your bladder, bowel and uterus in place, as well as helping to close the outlets of the bladder and bowel. The muscles also play a role in love-making – their contractions increase the pleasure for both you and your partner.

'I have only just realized that my pelvic floor muscles have been weakened – almost six months after the birth – because I have gone back to work and promptly caught a cold ... and every time I sneeze, I leak!'
Cecilia, mother of Joshua

These muscles and ligaments come under strain during pregnancy and childbirth so it is important to maintain their strength by exercises. The weight of your baby during pregnancy places a strain on the muscles, but the hormone relaxin often softens and stretches them. If you have any strain or weakness in these muscles, you may leak urine, particularly when you cough, laugh, sneeze or exercise.

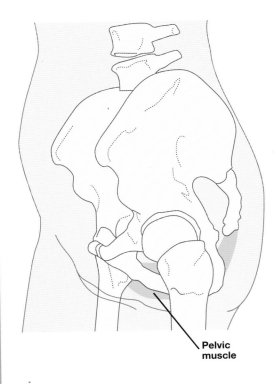

Pelvic muscle

Above: Regular exercise of pelvic floor muscles will help you control them during stage 2 of labour.

The importance of these exercises

Prolonged or repeated stretching of these muscles can result in permanent damage. If you ignore any weakness in your pelvic floor, you may develop conditions such as a prolapsed vagina, rectum, bladder or uterus. This is where the muscles fail to support the organs and start to 'drop', bulging into the vagina. This can result not only in urinary incontinence but also in lack of control over bowel movements. Surgery may be necessary to repair this.

When to start

There is no reason why you should not start doing these exercises as soon as you find out that you are pregnant. It is important to con-tinue them, not only during pregnancy but also after the baby is born, in order to regain your muscle tone. Do not leave it until after the birth because you will not be able to feel the mus-cles as well as you can now. In fact, all women should do these exercises throughout their lives to guard against stress incontinence (involuntary leakage of urine).

How to do the exercises

Follow the instructions (see box) and, in each case, relax the muscles quickly and then repeat the exercise. Try to combine the three exercises. Clench the muscles quickly several times and then do the exercises slowly again. Think about the positions of the different muscles and how they feel. Imagine the muscles as an elevator – rising three floors and stopping at each one. When they are on the top floor, lower them in stages, stopping at each floor! Repeat the exercises ten times, five times a day.

Pelvic floor exercises

Sit comfortably, with your back straight and your knees relaxed and held slightly apart.
- **Imagine that you are trying to avoid passing wind, or that you are 'holding on' to a desperate need to open your bowels. As you squeeze the muscles around your back passage you should feel the muscles move. Do not lift your buttocks or move your legs.**
- **Imagine you are sitting on the toilet to pass urine. Clench the muscles that you would use to stop the stream of urine and imagine drawing them up, like an elevator rising.**
- **Imagine that you are trying to grip a tampon in your vagina using your pelvic floor muscles.**

Check that you are doing the exercises properly by putting a finger into your vagina and feeling the muscles tighten as you clench. Develop an awareness of how your muscles feel when they are relaxed. This is important in the second stage of labour, when you are pushing out your baby. Tighten the muscles of your pelvic floor as you breathe in, and then, with each outward breath, slowly relax the muscles as much as possible.

Try to associate the exercise with another activity, for example when you have a drink or after you have passed water. It does not matter what position you are in – you could be standing, sitting, squatting or lying down. The great thing about these exercises is that you can do them anywhere and at any time and no one else will be any the wiser.

Emotional after-effects

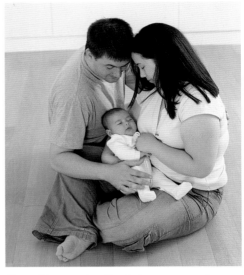

In the first few days, you may experience a range of emotions, from relief and elation to fear and exhaustion. Some women feel guilty because they could not follow their birth plan. Others are tired, uncomfortable because of stitches, and need time to get to know their baby. It is normal to have a sense of unreality, as well as feelings of inadequacy or anxiety.

Above: Time spent getting to know your newborn will help you bond as a family.

True story

Post-birth anxiety

'I have a fear of surgery and wanted minimal intervention, but the midwife realized my baby was breech at 39 weeks. My waters broke just before my due date and when I rang the hospital I was told to go in as soon as possible. A scan revealed that my baby was still bottom-first, and I was given a choice: natural or caesarean. I was terrified, but opted for a caesarean because I thought it might be safer.

'My husband Jim watched the operation and saw our son Jake being born. But as more and more doctors and nurses came into the room, we realized something was not right. Jake was grey, lifeless and not breathing. He had an Apgar score of just 1 and was clinging to life, with a weak heartbeat. The doctors whisked him off to the neonatal unit. We were distraught, waiting for news.

'After three days, Jake was taken off the ventilator and after five days he was back on the ward with me. Two days later we went home. He is now strong, healthy and happy, and I feel so grateful to the hospital staff. It had never crossed my mind that my baby would not be completely healthy. It took Jim and me quite a while to come to terms with being parents and to feel confident. I admit there were days when we would feel very low for no apparent reason. But overall, we just felt so lucky that our little man made it through.'

Karen, mother of Jake

Emotional after-effects **Common questions**

Q It is three weeks since I had my baby, and I am feeling really down – I keep bursting into tears for no apparent reason. Could I have post-natal depression?

A Adjusting to motherhood brings a range of emotions. Feeling sad, anxious, irritable, tired and lethargic can be signs of post-natal depression (PND). Every mother will have some days when these feelings come to the fore, and this is normal. However, if most of your days are like this, or if you notice that your low moods are becoming more frequent, talk to your midwife, health visitor or doctor. Post-natal depression can occur at any time during the first year after a baby's birth. As soon as it is diagnosed, appropriate support and treatment can begin, after which women almost always recover quickly.

Q I love my baby, but I cannot get over the disappointment of having her by caesarean.

A Disappointment and a sense of loss over the way your labour might have been are very common feelings. In the run-up to the birth it is natural to have hopes and expectations, and if they are unfulfilled, it is natural to feel sadness, anger, disappointment, even failure. In the post-natal period, there may be little time to air these feelings, leaving you with a sense of confusion and frustration when they do not fade away. Talk to your midwife, health visitor or doctor. Finding out the reasons for your caesarean might help you come to terms with it, and it may be helpful to look at your notes with your midwife.

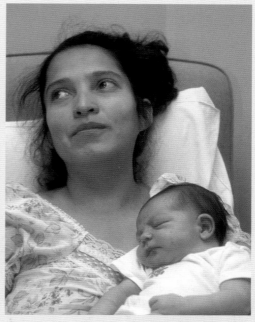

Above: You may suffer mood swings, experiencing emotions such as joy, anxiety, fear and excitement.

Q I had my first baby six weeks ago and I found the birth very traumatic. Is it normal to feel like this? My husband says I should be grateful that we have a healthy baby.

A You are certainly not alone in the way that you feel. Many women are like you, but feel guilty that they keep dwelling on the birth when everyone else is focusing on the baby. For some women, childbirth can be very traumatic and not the joyful experience they hoped for. It is essential that you explore why you feel so traumatized by the birth. Many hospital units have a facility where women have the chance to reflect on the birth, as the benefits of doing this are now widely recognized.

Caesarean recovery

If you were in a fit and healthy condition before the birth, you are likely to recover quickly after a caesarean, although you will feel a bit wobbly to begin with. However, problems can occur if you do not have enough rest and support afterwards. You may find that being unable to perform such a simple task as lifting or holding your baby is particularly frustrating. Ask your midwife for advice.

Your midwife can show you different positions that may help, for example, placing a pillow on your lap, lying down or holding your baby under your arm to feed him. It is important to continue your pelvic floor exercises (see page 112) because the muscles lost tone during your pregnancy and will have been affected by the operation. However, you should avoid strenuous activities (including driving, lifting and housework) for the first six weeks. Make the most of any help offered because you will need time to recover from the operation, as well as having a new baby to look after.

Five tips for conserving energy after a **caesarean**

A caesarean, like any other operation, will drain your energy reserves and, in addition, you will have a new baby to look after. Until you are fully recovered, it pays to make your life as easy as you can.

1 Delegate as much as possible. Accept all serious offers of help and suggest specific jobs, such as vacuuming or taking older children to playgroup.

2 If something does not need doing straight away, put it off until the following day or, better still, week.

3 Have somewhere for your baby to sleep and a set of nappy-changing equipment upstairs and downstairs to save journeys. A table at the right height for nappy changing saves any bending.

4 Take a nap during the day when your baby is sleeping.

5 You probably won't have much of an appetite after the operation. Eat little and often to maintain your energy.

Caesarean recovery **Common questions**

Q Will I be in much pain after a caesarean?
A Pain varies from person to person and can be severe at first, but adequate pain relief will help to speed your recovery. Some hospitals use patient-controlled analgesia (PCA), where you give yourself pain relief through a machine with a device to prevent overdoses. In the days afterwards, some women use a TENS machine or the breathing techniques that they learned for labour (see page 58). In a couple of days, paracetamol or anti-inflammatories may provide sufficient pain relief. Tell staff if the pain does not diminish, or gets worse, as this could indicate an infection that needs antibiotics.

Q Can I breastfeed my baby after a caesarean section?
A You will be able to breastfeed as soon as you feel ready. Anaesthetic drugs cause no problems. Your milk usually comes in around the third day, although it sometimes takes a little longer. Initially, the colostrum provides your baby with all he needs. Experiment until you find a comfortable position – your midwife can advise you. It may be easier to feed your baby in bed.

Q How long does it take to recover?
A Full recovery after a caesarean birth takes anything between a month and two years, but the average is about six months. Your scar will be red at first, then pink, and finally it will fade to white or silver, possibly remaining numb for

Right: Lying on your side in bed is a comfortable position for breastfeeding after a caesarean section.

several months. However, physical healing is only part of the process. An emergency caesarean tests your reserves of courage far more than a normal birth. Many women are overwhelmed by fear. This fear does not always disappear once the crisis is over, and you may experience a delayed reaction.

Q I had an emergency caesarean section with my first child. Is this likely to be the case with my second?
A 'Once a Caesar, always a Caesar' is an old wives' tale. It depends on the circumstances – for example, fetal distress is unlikely to happen twice. Regardless of the reason for their first caesarean, more than two-thirds of women go on to have a normal birth. If the operation was uncomplicated, with a bikini-line scar, your care next time would probably be little different from any other woman in labour.

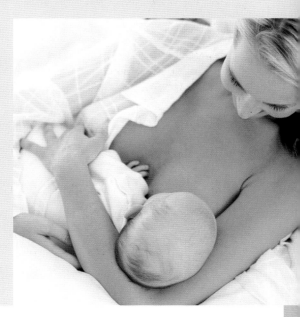

Father and baby

It can be hard for a new father to feel involved in the day-to-day care of a new baby, especially as, on the surface, not much may have changed for him. He may well still be getting up and going out to work, and he may lack confidence initially when it comes to handling the baby. In some cases, a mother can be so focused on the baby that the father hardly gets a look in.

Five ways for fathers to **get involved**

Involving the father will not only give you some quiet time but will also help him to become closer to your baby. There are a number of things that he can do.

1 Bathe the baby – this is the perfect way to end the day and can be great fun.
2 Schedule regular 'father time'– take over for a couple of hours in the evening while you get some rest before the night feeds.
3 Put the baby in a sling or into her pram and take her out for some fresh air.
4 Help out with night feeds – if you can express milk.
5 Massage the baby by gently rubbing baby oil into her body in a warm room.

Give him a chance to learn with you

For men to be successful fathers, they have to be given the chance to get involved. This can be hard, especially if you feel that you are the only one who really understands your baby. However, you have only come to know her ways through trial and error, and your partner needs to be given the same opportunity. Stand back and let him make his own mistakes. If you cannot watch him without trying to correct him, walk away.

Make some family time

As you and your partner become absorbed in the practical day-to-day elements of child care and running a home, it can be easy to forget your parenting role. Remember that you are a family. Make time to do things together, whether it is enjoying a day out or simply both being there at bath time occasionally. Enjoying family time is what having children is all about – and your child will begin to understand that you are a team.

Fathers are very important

Allowing your partner to be a hands-on father brings benefits to the whole family. Your baby will enjoy even more love and attention and will thrive from experiencing different parenting styles. At the same time, your partner will relish the opportunity to get to know his baby and to explore his new role. Studies have shown that fathers who become more involved in the day-to-day baby care tend to be much closer to their children.

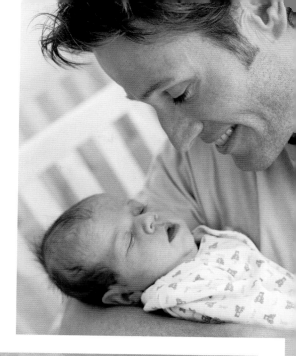

Although research suggests that fathers parent babies in a very similar way to mothers, men also offer some unique and irreplaceable qualities. Fathers often develop a special skill, perhaps bathing the baby, getting her back to sleep, or doing a quick nappy change. So try not to see your partner as just an assistant – instead acknowledge that he has a special role in your child's life that will grow and develop as your child grows older.

Right: A father has a special role in a child's life, so give him the space to get involved.

True
story

A father's point of view

'It is great being a new dad. Every day is full of surprises and when you have never had a child before you do not know what to expect. Before Matteo was born, I would speak to different people about what it was like to have a baby and most of the comments, although made in a joking way, were quite negative. But I think it has all been beautiful, not difficult at all. Even though Matteo wakes in the night, it is worth getting up to give him a cuddle.

'Now that I am back at work, my day starts with Matteo waking me at 6.30am. Sometimes he comes in beside us for a cuddle, and I spend a few minutes with him before making my breakfast. When I go in to say goodbye, Sylvia and Matteo are usually asleep. It is such a lovely picture to have in your head when you leave the house in the morning.

'Sylvia says I am a natural dad, and I think I am too! It is really important for me to give Matteo and Sylvia all of my energy. Before Matteo was born, I worked five days a week, often until 10pm, but I do not want to be a dad who is not around for his children. So I have decided to work four days a week and top up my salary by giving private tuition on a couple of evenings. This leaves so much more time to spend as a family. Matteo is changing every day and I do not want to miss it.'

Vincent, father of Matteo

Going home

Most mothers normally leave hospital within a day or two of the birth, although you may stay longer if there are any problems. The prospect of caring for your baby on your own can seem daunting, but your midwife will visit you for up to ten days, and longer if necessary. When she signs you off, the health visitor will take over.

Make rest a priority for at least 21 days after the birth. You will want visitors, but the most welcome ones will admire your baby, tell you how clever you are, drop off a little present – and leave! Unless they are genuinely helpful, and you get on very well, having relatives to stay can be exhausting.

Although you may feel fine at first, you will soon run out of energy, so rest whenever you can. If you have used up your reserves of emotional energy by trying to do too much, something minor and temporary – such as your baby waking frequently at night or a minor feeding problem – can become blown up out of all proportion.

Crying

Newborn babies cry more than most – sometimes up to three or four hours a day. It is not always easy to know why a baby cries, and this can be hugely frustrating for a new mother. Crying is a new baby's way of telling you that something is wrong. He does not know exactly what the problem is, only that he is uncomfortable or in pain. It is left to you to find out what is wrong (see box).

Why is my baby crying?

Ask yourself the following questions.
- **Is he ill?** If your baby shows signs of not eating normally, or has diarrhoea or a raised temperature, he could be unwell. Consult your doctor if you are concerned.
- **Is he hungry?** Babies have small tummies and need frequent feeds in the early days. If it is two to three hours since his last feed, hunger could be the problem.
- **Is he tired?** Babies can get irritable when they need to sleep but have trouble settling.
- **Is he wet or dirty?** If your baby needs a nappy change, this could be why he is crying.

- **Is he uncomfortable?** Check all over for an obvious cause of discomfort, such as a finger caught in his shawl, overly tight clothes, being propped up instead of lying down.
- **Is he too hot or too cold?** Young babies cannot regulate their temperatures easily and quickly become overheated or chilly.
- **Is he lonely?** Your baby needs regular physical contact from you. Give him a cuddle to reassure him that you are nearby.
- **Is he bored?** New babies love stimulation, so make sure he is positioned where he can see plenty going on.

Bathing

A new washing up bowl is perfectly adequate for bathing a new baby. Put about 6 cm (2–3 in) of water in the bath, testing the temperature with your elbow or wrist to make sure that it is just warm. Some babies love a bath, others hate it, but a quick dip will suffice. Never leave your baby alone in the bath.

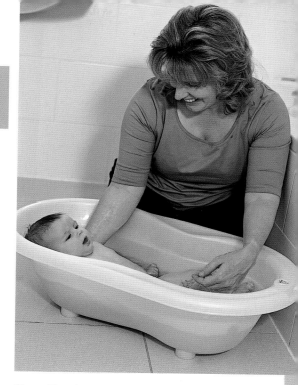

Above: Test the water temperature before bathing a baby, and never leave a baby alone in a bath.

Top and tailing

In the first few days, your baby will not get very dirty. It is enough to bathe him about twice a week and, in the meantime, to 'top and tail' him.
• Have everything you need to hand: changing mat, bowl of lukewarm water, cotton wool, small, soft towel, clean nappy and clean clothes.
• Lay your baby on his changing mat on a nappy or towel and remove his clothes.
• If his eyes are sticky, wipe one eye with moistened cotton wool, wiping from the inside of the eyelid outwards. Then wipe the other eye with fresh cotton wool.
• Wipe around his ears, over his face and neck, under his chin and then over his hands. Use fresh cotton wool each time and pat the area dry with a towel, making sure that no dampness is left in the creases.
• Change the nappy and put on clean clothes.
• Don't bathe the cord unless it becomes sticky, in which case use cotton wool and water. It will separate more quickly if it is allowed to dry in the air, with the nappy slightly folded over it.

Nappy rash

Nappy rash usually occurs if a soiled nappy is left on for too long. A baby's stool is full of bacteria, which react with the urine to form ammonia, irritating the skin and leaving it red and sore. To avoid nappy rash, adopt the following procedures.
• Change your baby's nappy whenever it becomes wet or dirty.
• Clean the whole nappy area thoroughly (from front to back with girls) using cotton wool and lukewarm tap water.
• Dry the area thoroughly before applying a thin layer of barrier cream.

Feeding

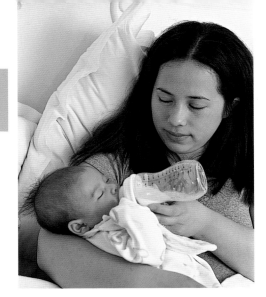

Above: As with breastfeeding, bottle-feeding should be given on demand, when your baby is hungry.

Breastfeeding is undoubtedly better for your baby's health and development, and 98 per cent of women are able to breastfeed. Nevertheless, it is not always possible, either because of a medical condition or because the mother is just not comfortable with it. Don't feel guilty if you don't want to breastfeed: formula milk will meet your baby's dietary needs, and there is no reason why she should not thrive on it.

Breastfeeding

Breast milk is produced on a basis of supply and demand. For the first two or three days, until your milk comes in, your breasts produce colostrum (a thick, creamy substance, packed with antibodies to protect your baby from infections and disease). The more your baby feeds at the breast, the more milk you will produce. The milk is made up of thirst-quenching foremilk, followed by the thicker hind milk.

Bottle-feeding

Bottle-feeding should also be on demand, and your baby will let you know when she is hungry. You may find that she will take more at some feeds than others and that she will feed more frequently at certain times of the day. It takes longer for babies to digest formula milk so they do tend to go longer between feeds. A newborn baby will probably take six or seven feeds in 24 hours and, for the first two or three days, will be taking 60 ml (2 fl oz) at a feed.

Five tips on bottle-feeding

Hygiene is very important when bottle-feeding because milk residue is an ideal breeding ground for bacteria.

1 Wash bottles and teats thoroughly in warm soapy water, using a bottlebrush.
2 Wash your hands thoroughly before making up feeds.
3 Do not store prepared bottles of formula milk in a refrigerator for more than 24 hours after they have reached room temperature.
4 Do not keep the contents of a bottle for more than an hour after your baby has finished drinking.
5 Do not increase the amount of powder in the feed just because your baby seems hungry. Not making up the feed properly can be very dangerous.

Feeding **Common questions**

Q When is the best time to feed my baby?

A The best time to start feeding is when your baby is calm, comfortable and alert. If she is fretful, try to soothe her first by rocking her. If you are breastfeeding and find she is too sleepy to feed, put her to the breast as often as you can to try to encourage her to begin rooting (searching for the nipple). If she is deeply asleep, look for hunger cues, such as licking her lips or rooting, and if you need to wake her, try tickling her feet gently.

Q For how long should I feed my baby?

A Always let your baby determine the length of a feed. A newborn's tummy is only about the size of a walnut, so she will need frequent feeds – perhaps as many as 10–12 a day for the first few weeks. When she has finished, she will let go of your nipple or the teat on the bottle and drift off to sleep. If you are breastfeeding, it is a good idea to alternate breasts with each feed to ensure that each is drained in turn.

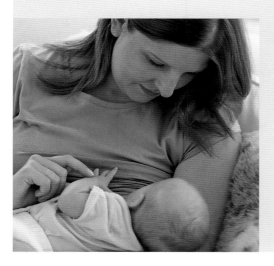

Q What is the best position for me to be in when I'm breastfeeding?

A Always take a couple of minutes to make sure you are comfortable and relaxed before beginning to feed your baby. Have everything you need within reach – the phone, a glass of water, a book. Sitting upright is the easiest position to start with. Have a pillow behind your back and place another across your lap to bring you baby level with your breasts. You may also find it easier if you have something on which to rest your arm, as your baby may be feeding for some time.

Q I am breastfeeding. How can I be sure my baby is latching on properly?

A When your baby latches on, her mouth should be wide open, to take in both your nipple and your areola (the darker area around the nipple). If she only latches on to your nipple, she will not be able to feed properly and you may get sore nipples. When she latches on properly, your nipple will be up towards the roof of her mouth, with her chin pressed into your breast. You will see her jaw moving slowly and rhythmically, and you may feel a slight drawing sensation as the milk flows. When she comes off the breast, your nipple will be slightly elongated.

Left: Breast milk is the best nutrition for your baby, but not all mothers are able or happy to breastfeed.

Sleeping

On average, your newborn baby will sleep for a total of 18 hours of 24 – but he will still keep you busy. He has developed his own sleeping pattern in the womb, so it is unrealistic to expect him to follow your sleeping pattern immediately now that he has been born.

Newborn babies are not aware of night and day, but sleep whenever they feel the need. They also have a short sleep cycle, moving from deep sleep to light sleep about every 20 minutes, compared with 90 minutes in an adult. Furthermore, newborn babies cannot sleep for 12 hours without feeding because their stomachs are so small.

Encouraging good sleeping habits

In the early days, there will be no routine. During the period just after the birth, it is a good idea to allow yourself to be led by your baby. Sleeping when he sleeps, including during the day, will give you a chance to catch up on some much-needed rest. At this time you should be concentrating as much as possible on feeding your baby and sleeping – other things can wait.

Some women like to put their baby down to sleep while he is still awake. In this way, he will learn to go off to sleep by himself and he will find it easier to settle when he wakes in the night. Your baby will soon learn to distinguish between night and day and you will gradually be able to establish a routine.

Sleep safety

Follow these guidelines to make sure that your baby sleeps safely.

- Place your baby on his back, with his feet at the bottom of his basket or cot, without a cot bumper.
- Keep the room temperature at about 18°C and place two blankets (not folded) no higher than his shoulders. Do not cover his head with any sort of hat.
- His hands and feet will often feel cold, so judge your baby's temperature by feeling his abdomen.
- Never put him next to a radiator or heater, or give him a hot-water bottle.
- Never let anyone smoke around your baby.
- Keep him in your room for the first six months, but only let him share your bed when you are breastfeeding.
- Never allow him into your bed if you smoke, take drugs or have been drinking alcohol.
- Never sleep on a sofa with your baby.

Sleeping **Common questions**

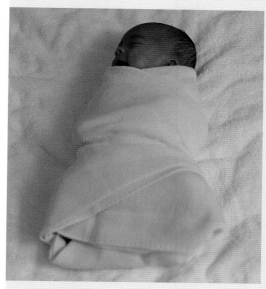

Above: Swaddling can make a newborn feel more secure, but take care not to overheat the baby.

Q Should I swaddle my newborn when he sleeps?

A Newborn babies are not accustomed to open spaces, and some may find the movement of their limbs alarming. Swaddling – wrapping them in a sheet with their arms tucked in – can prevent this. Make sure that the swaddling is only one layer thick and does not cover the head, and that you place your baby on his back to sleep. It is important not to overheat your baby.

Q My neighbour says her daughter slept right through the night at six weeks. Is this really possible?

A Some mothers boast that their babies are sleeping 'through the night', but what do they really mean? A six-week-old is incapable of sleeping for 12 hours without feeding, so your neighbour probably means her daughter is sleeping from 11pm to 5am – long enough for the mother to get a good night's rest, but not really sleeping through the night. Most babies are six months old before they can go without a night feed.

Q My baby is wakeful during the night, leaving me exhausted during the day. What can I do?

A Don't worry if your baby is wakeful – you just need to work out how best to manage. Rest whenever you can during the day and go to bed early. This alone will not make up for the broken nights, so share the load with your partner. If you are breastfeeding you could express some milk for your partner to give to the baby after you have gone to bed. Power naps can help to 'take the edge' off the exhaustion. Don't forget to eat and drink in order to keep up your energy levels.

index

acknowledgements

Hamlyn would like to thank *Practical Parenting*'s midwife, **Anne Richley**, for her invaluable help with the questions and answers and for checking information and pictures. Thanks also to **Mara Lee** for her very helpful input.

Executive Editor **Jane McIntosh**
General Editor **Anna Southgate**
Project Editor **Alice Bowden, Fiona Robertson**
Executive Art Editor **Darren Southern**
Designer **Ginny Zeal**
Production Assistant **Nosheen Shan**
Picture Researcher **Aruna Mathar**

Alamy/Jennie Hart 30. Corbis UK Ltd/94, 117, Marc Asnin 108, Baci/Stephen Dupont 32, The Cover Story/Floris Leeuwenberg 34, Owen Franken 58, Janet Jarman 97, Louis Quail 4 centre bottom, 80, David Stoecklein 29, Vince Streano 44, LWA/Dann Tardif 6, Zefa/H.Schmid 4 top, 8, Larry Williams and Associates 3. Getty Images/Tom Grill 4 bottom, 100, Charles Gullung 24. Octopus Publishing Group Limited/Ruth Jenkins 17 left, Peter Myers 17 right, Daniel Panbourne 38, 69, 84 left, 84 right, 85 top left, 85 top right, 85 bottom, Adrian Pope 7, 19, 114 top, Peter Pugh Cook 23, 36 top right, Russell Sadur 1, 104, 121, 122, 123, 125, Gareth Sambidge 39. Angela Hampton/Family Life Picture Library 4 centre top, 18, 40, 42, 49, 55, 72, 115. Jupiterimages/Andersen Ross 20. Photolibrary Group/Phototake Inc./Brad Nelson 14, Purestock 102, Bananastock 119, Photodisc 12 top, 12 bottom. Science Photo Library/Ian Hooton 4 centre, 60, MIDIRS/Ruth Jenkinson 75.

To subscribe to *Practical Parenting* magazine call 0845 6767778 or click on **www.ipcmedia.com**